EMPHYSEMA

Edited by **Ravi Mahadeva**

Emphysema
Edited by Ravi Mahadeva

Published by InTech
Janeza Trdine 9, 51000 Rijeka, Croatia

Publishing Process Manager Molly Kaliman

Technical Editor Teodora Smiljanic

Cover Designer InTech Design Team

Additional hard copies can be obtained from orders@intechopen.com

Emphysema, Edited by Ravi Mahadeva
p. cm.
ISBN 978-953-51-0433-9

For EU product safety concerns:
IN TECH d.o.o., Prolaz Marije Krucifikse Kozulić 3, 51000 Rijeka, Croatia,
info@intechopen.com or visit our website at intechopen.com.

Meet the editor

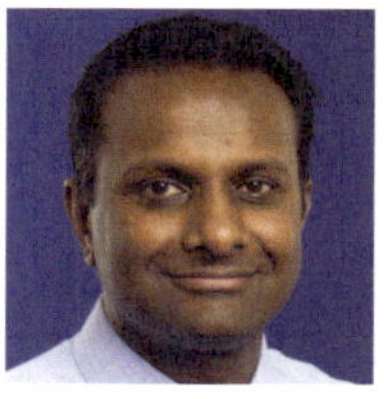

Dr Ravi Mahadeva is Director of the Cambridge COPD Centre and Clinical Director for Respiratory Medicine, Cambridge University Hospitals Foundation Trust and Associate Lecturer, Department of Medicine, University of Cambridge. He trained in pulmonary medicine in London and Cambridge, UK, and was a recipient of a Wellcome Trust Advanced Clinical Fellowship to work on the pathogenesis of emphysema at Washington University, St Louis and Harvard Medical School, USA. He was awarded the prestigious European Respiratory Society COPD research award 2004.

Contents

Preface

The last decade has seen the emergence of COPD as a major health problem world-wide. The recognition of this has stimulated the biomedical community to actively research in this area, towards understanding the pathogenesis of this devastating disease. This book contains a mixture of summaries of complex molecular pathogenic mechanisms, emerging new clinical entities and novel treatments. The book begins with sections on pathogenesis, innate immunity, anti-proteinase function and a review of the relationship between hypothesis, basic science and the development of a related treatment. These chapters are followed by description of the newly recognized association between pulmonary fibrosis within COPD and state-of-the art descriptions of novel bronchoscopic treatments and new strategies for the management of the common clinical problem of air leaks. It is currently an exciting time in COPD, and it is hoped that this book will stimulate further interest in this hitherto relatively neglected disease.

Dr Ravi Mahadeva
Director of the Cambridge COPD Centre and Clinical Director for Respiratory Medicine,
Cambridge University Hospitals Foundation Trust and Associate Lecturer,
Department of Medicine, University of Cambridge
United Kingdom

1

Pathogenic Mechanisms in Emphysema: From Protease Anti–Protease Imbalance to Apoptosis

Raja T. Abboud
Division of Respiratory Medicine,
University of British Columbia at Vancouver General Hospital,
Seymour Health Centre Vancouver,
Canada

1. Introduction

In 1963, Laurel and Erickson reported their discovery of severe α_1-antitrypsin (AAT) deficiency and its association with emphysema (Laurell & Erickson, 1963). Soon after, Gross and coworkers reported that emphysema was induced in rats by the intratracheal instillation of a proteolytic enzyme (Gross et al.,1965). These findings led to the proteolytic hypothesis of emphysema (Janoff, 1985) which considers that emphysema develops as a result of the smoking-induced release of proteolytic enzymes from the increased number of neutrophils and macrophages in the lung. Proteolysis of lung connective tissue (more specifically elastin) occurs because the released proteases may not be fully inhibited by antiproteases, resulting in emphysema. However, although proteolysis may have a significant pathogenic role particularly in AAT deficiency, other pathogenic mechanism, such as oxidants either from inhaled smoke or from inflammatory cells, inflammation, T lymphocyte cell mediated immunity, and apoptosis have a significant pathogenic role (MacNee, a2005).

This chapter, based on a previous review article (Abboud & Vimalanathan, 2008), updated and revised following a Pub-Med search, and will cover protease-antiprotease imbalance and apoptosis, as pathogenic mechanisms in emphysema. The pathogenic role of oxidants, inflammatory cells, and cell mediated immunity will be covered in other chapters.

2. Protease-antiprotease imbalance in severe antitrypsin deficiency

The hypothesis that the main pathogenic mechanism in emphysema in severe AAT deficiency is due to protease-antiprotease , is well supported by evidence since AAT is the main inhibitor of neutrophil elastase. Since this topic will be discussed in detail in another chapter, this paragraph will serve as a brief introduction. In severe AAT deficiency, anti-elastase protection in the lung interstitium and alveolar space is markedly decreased in proportion to the decreased plasma levels to about 15-20 % of normal, and does not fully protect the lung against released neutrophil elastase. Neutrophil elastase is a potent elastolytic enzyme, which induces emphysema when injected intratracheally in experimental animals (Janoff et al.,1977; Senior et al,1977). Smoking increases the number of neutrophils in the lung, and induces the release of neutrophil elastase (Fera et al., 1986; Abboud et al. 1986). The released neutrophil elastase may not be fully inhibited by the severely deficient AAT levels leading to proteolytic activity and the development of emphysema. The positive correlation between increased leucocyte elastase concentration and severity of emphysema in patients with severe AAT deficiency, supports a pathogenic role for neutrophil elastase in AAT deficient emphysema (Kidokoro et al.,1977).

3. Protease antiprotease imbalance in copd without severe antitrypsin deficiency

In contrast, in smokers with COPD without AAT deficiency , there is less evidence to support protease antiprotease imbalance as a pathogenic mechanism in emphysema, compared with AAT deficient smokers, because there is no definitive evidence of severe antiprotease deficiency to lead to unopposed proteolysis in the lung. Smoking may cause a protease-antiprotease imbalance in the lung by decreasing the functional activity of AAT and other protease inhibitors in the lung interstitium and "alveolar" lining fluid, and by increasing the amount of elastolytic proteases released in the lung. Some studies reported that smokers had decreased anti-elastase activity of AAT in BAL, compared with nonsmokers (Gadek et al., 1979; Carp et al., 1982). However, this reported degree of inactivation was not confirmed by later studies (Stone et al.,1983; Boudier et al., 1983; Abboud et al., 1985).

3.1 Studies evaluating neutrophil elastase in emphysema

Cigarette smoking can induce the release of neutrophil elastase (NE) in BAL of healthy volunteers (Fera et al.,1986), and intense smoking can acutely increase plasma NE levels (Abboud et al., 1986). NE released in the lung may be taken up and internalized by alveolar macrophages (AM) (Campbell et al., 1979) . A study evaluating BAL in 28 patients with COPD supported a role for NE and protease-antiprotease imbalance by showing that NE levels in BAL correlated directly and BAL anti-elastase activity correlated inversely with emphysema, assessed by CT scan and carbon monoxide diffusing capacity (Fujita et al.,1990). Another study of older volunteers reported increased levels of NE in AM of smokers with CT scan evidence of emphysema (Betsuyaku et al.,1995), suggesting that NE release in the lung and its uptake by AM could have been a pathogenic factor in emphysema. NE bound to elastin may continue to degrade elastin despite the presence of active AAT in the surrounding medium (Morrison et al., 1990). All these findings support a potential role for NE in the development of human emphysema, despite the lack of severe inactivation of AAT in the lung. The pathogenic role of NE was also confirmed in a mouse NE-knockout exposed to cigarette smoke, where the resulting emphysema was reduced by 59% compared with control smoke-exposed mice (Shapiro et al., 2003). This was not all a direct effect of the absence of NE activity, but partly secondary to decreased macrophage recruitment in the absence of NE; it could be also partly due to the lack of degradation by NE of tissue inhibitors of metalloproteases which inhibit macrophage elastase activity.

3.2 Potential role of macrophage proteases in emphysema

It is likely that macrophage proteases have a pathogenic role for in human emphysema. Investigators reported that young smokers dying accidentally had an increased number of macrophages in the respiratory bronchioles (Niewoehner et al., 1974), in the same region where centrilobular emphysema develops in smokers without AAT deficiency. Morphometry of resected human lungs indicated that the extent of emphysema was directly related to the numbers of AM but not neutrophils (Finkelstein et al., 1995). These two studies suggested a potential role of macrophages in emphysema. Elastolysis by AM *in vitro* was not inhibited by AAT, while that of neutrophils was inhibited (Chapman et al., 1984; Chapman & Stone 1984). This finding supported a pathogenic role for AM elastolytic enzymes in emphysema, since these AM enzymes would not be inhibited by AAT, the major protease inhibitor in plasma and interstitial fluid. Subsequently, investigators demonstrated several elastolytic enzymes in human AM: cathepsins L and S (Reilly et al., 1989; Reilly et al.,1991; Shi et al.,1992), the matrix metalloproteases (MMPs) MMP-2 and MMP-9, previously termed 72 & 92 kDa collagenases respectively (Senior et al., 1991) and MMP-12 also named macrophage metallo-elastase (Shapiro et al., 1993). In addition, interstitial collagenase or MMP1, a non-elastolytic enzyme , induced emphysema in transgenic mice expressing MMP1 (D'Armiento et al., 1992; Foronjy et al 2003), by degrading type III collagen (Shiomy et al., 2003).

Several studies support a pathogenic role for AM in human emphysema, by comparing findings in subjects with and without emphysema Cultured AM from patients with emphysema showed increased elastolytic activity compared with that of AM from patients with bronchitis or other lung diseases (Muley et al., 1994). In a study of 34 healthy smokers (mean age 46 yr), there was a significantly greater AM cell counts in BAL in those with emphysema by computed tomography (CT) compared to those without emphysema; this finding indicated a greater AM elastase load in the lungs in those with emphysema, since the AM elastolytic activity/cell was similar in the two groups (Abboud et al., 1998). AM obtained by BAL from 10 emphysema patients, had increased expression of MMP9 and MMP1, when compared with 10 matched controls (Finlay et al., 1997). Emphysematous lung tissue had significantly higher levels of MMP9 and MMP2 compared with control non-involved lung tissue; and showed elastolytic activity corresponding to MMP2 and MMP9 (Ohnishi et al.,1998). A study using immunohistochemistry of lung tissue, showed increases in MMP1, MMP2, MMP8, and MMP9 in lung tissue from COPD patients compared with controls (Segura-Valdez et al., 2000). There was increased expression of MMP1 in the lungs of patients with emphysema (Imai et al., 2001); however, the MMP1 was localized to the type II epithelial cells and not macrophages.

Cigarette smoke induced emphysema in mice requires MMP12; mice homozygous for a knockout of the MMP12 gene, in contrast to controls, did not develop emphysema in response to cigarette smoke exposure (Hautamaki et al., 1997). However, MMP12 is much more highly expressed in mice compared with humans. A study in COPD patients reported that the number of AM in BAL expressing MMP12 and the level of MMP12 expression was higher in COPD than in controls (Molet et al., 2005). Increased MMP levels by ELISA in induced sputum from 26 stable COPD patients were significantly higher than healthy smokers, never smokers, and former smokers (Demedst et al., 2006); in addition MMP12 enzyme activity in the COPD subjects was markedly increased compared with non-smokers. These two studies support a potential pathogenic role for MMP12 in human emphysema.

Smoking and pro-inflammatory stimuli can induce message expression of AM elastases and proteases, which could lead to protease-antiprotease imbalance. Smokers have increased expression of cathepsin L in AM compared to non-smokers (Takahashi et al.,1993), and also increased activity of cathepsin S in AM lysates (Reilly et al., 1991). Pro-inflammatory mediators induce expression of MMPs, such as the marked increase in mRNA for MMP12 in cultured AM by lipopolysaccharide (LPS) (Shapiro et al., 1993). TNF-α and IL-1β increased expression of MMP9 by human macrophages without increasing its inhibitor, tissue inhibitor of metalloprotease (TIMP1) (Saren et al., 1996); these two cytokines , which are increased in COPD, may thus lead to a protease-antiprotease imbalance between MMP9 and its inhibitor. The release of TNF-α in mice by cigarette smoke was dependent on MMP-12 (Churg et al., 2003), and was abolished in MMP12 knockout mice; TNF-α accounted for 70% of the smoke induced emphysema in the mouse (Churg et al., 2004). In-vitro studies showed that AM from patients with COPD released more MMP9 than AM from healthy smokers, and MMP9 release was increased by IL-1β, LPS, and cigarette smoke solution (Russell et al., 2002a) . The same investigator reported that MMPs, cysteine and serine proteases contributed to the in-vitro elastolysis by human AM during the 72 hr evaluation (Russell et al., 2002b), indicating the difficulty in implicating a specific protease in lung destruction.

A recent study (Omachi et al.,2011) evaluated plasma MMP9 levels in relation to progression of emphysema over a period of one year, in 126 subjects with severe AAT deficiency who were on placebo treatment in a clinical trial evaluating AAT augmentation therapy. They found that higher baseline plasma MMP-9 levels were associated with lower values of FEV_1 and CO diffusing capacity (p=0.03), but not CT scan lung density. Moreover, MMP-9 levels predicted a decline in CO pulmonary diffusing capacity (p=0.04) and worsening lung density by CT scan (p=0.003). This relationship may not apply in human emphysema without severe AAT deficiency. A thorough and elaborate study evaluated the role of MMP9 in cigarette smoke induced emphysema in mice and humans (Atkinson et al., 2011); I will restrict my review to the human findings. Macrophage MMP-9 mRNA isolated by laser capture micro-dissection from 5 human lungs obtained at the time of lung transplantation were similar in areas of lung with and without emphysema. The investigators also enrolled subjects who had completed a National Lung Screening Trial and were free of cancer or an inflammatory or immune disorder into their emphysema biomarker study. Of these 38 had a CT scan emphysema index >10% and were considered to be "emphysema-sensitive", while 47 had an emphysema index of <5% and were "emphysema-resistant" controls. Circulating monocyte MMP9 mRNA showed a positive correlation with emphysema index for all subjects (p=0.02), and a more significant correlation in the "emphysema-sensitive" group (p-0.01), but there was no statistical difference in results between the two groups. There was no correlation of circulating monocyte MMP9 mRNA with the lung injury markers used, Clara cell secretory protein and surfactant protein-D. It would be interesting to check the correlation of emphysema extent with MMP9 plasma levels, which may be a better marker of MMP9 release in the lungs than levels in circulating monocytes.

In studies from my laboratory on alveolar macrophages (AM) lavaged from resected lung specimens, the level of mRNA expression of MMP1 in AM showed a significant positive correlation with the extent of emphysema by CT scan (Wallace et al., 2008). In addition, MMP12 mRNA expression was increased in current smokers vs ex-smokers, and there was there was a significant negative correlation between MMP12 gene expression and carbon monoxide diffusing capacity. These results support a pathogenic role for both MMP1 and MMP12 in human emphysema. A pathogenic role for cathepsin K in the development of emphysema was demonstrated in smoke-exposed guinea pigs compared with controls, and there were also data supporting increased expression of cathepsin K in lungs of emphysema patients (Golovatch et al., 2009).

Fig 1 is a diagram of potential mechanisms leading to protease antiprotease imbalance and emphysema.

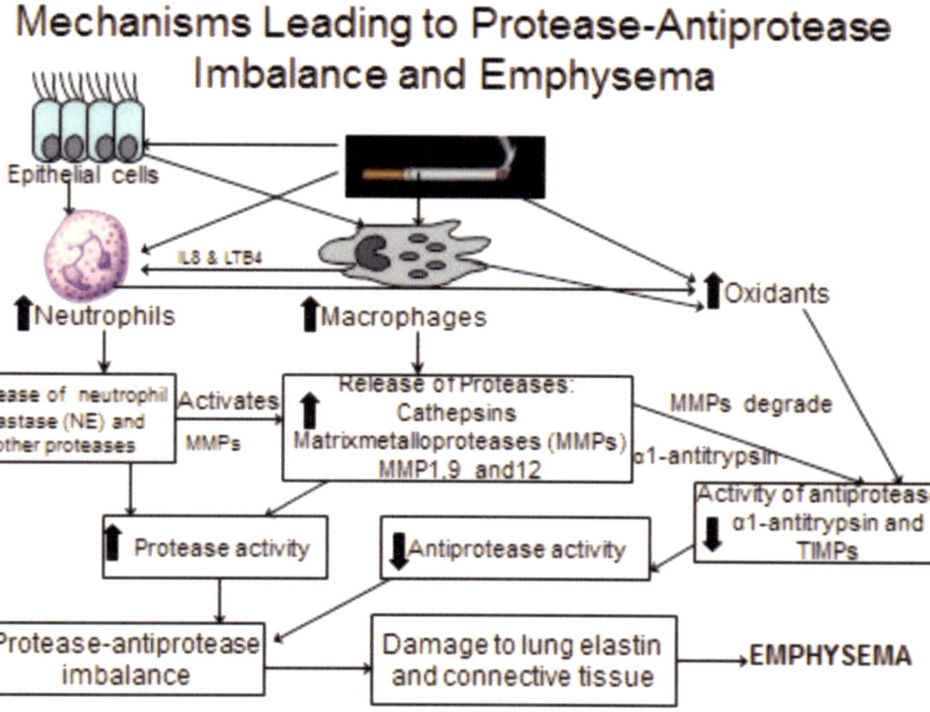

Fig. 1. Diagram showing the pathways leading to smoking-induced protease-antiprotease imbalance in the lung. (Reproduced from Abboud, R. , & Vimanalathan, S. (2008), with permission of the publisher, Int J Tuberc Lung Dis)

Smoking induces epithelial cells to produce cytokines which stimulate neutrophils and macrophages. Cigarette smoke also acts directly on neutrophils and macrophages to activate them . Cigarette smoke has oxidants which can inactivate antiproteases, in addition to antiprotease inactivation by oxidants released by macrophages and neutrophils.

The stimulated neutrophils and macrophages release proteolytic enzymes. Neutrophil elastase can activate MMPs, while MMPs can inactivate α_1-antitrypsin. Not shown in the diagram, is the role of MMP-12 in releasing TNF-α, which amplifies the inflammatory reaction. These processes lead to a protease-antiprotease imbalance, which can degrade lung elastin and connective tissue; if sustained, this will lead to emphysema.

3.3 Role of polymorphisms in MMPs

An MMP polymorphism (C-15621) was associated with emphysema by CT scan in one Japanese study (Minematsu et al., 2001) and with upper lobe emphysema in another Japanese study (Ito et al., 2005), and with COPD in a Chinese population (Zhou et al., 2004).

A study from Russia evaluated gene polymorphisms of G(-1607)GG of MMP1, C(-1562)T of MMP9, and A(-82)G of MMP12, and found the frequencies did not differ significantly between 318 COPD patients compared with 319 healthy controls (Korytina et al., 2008). However, the (-1562)T allele of MMP9 was significantly higher in the Global Initiative for Chronic Obstructive Lung Disease (GOLD) stage IV COPD than in stages II and III, indicating that this allele predisposed to severe disease; it also predisposed to early onset of COPD (age < 55 yr).

A multicentre European study determined 26 single nucleotide polymorphisms (SNP)s, covering reported SNP variations, in MMPs- 1, 9 and 12 from 977 COPD patients and 876 non-diseased smokers of European descent and evaluated their association with disease singly and in haplotype combinations (Haq., et al. 2010). They used logistic regression to adjust for age, gender, centre, and smoking history. They reported that the common A-A haplotypes of two SNPs in MMP-12 (rs652438 and rs2276109), were associated with severe or very severe disease (GOLD Stages III and IV) ($p = 0.0039$).

This review has focused on neutrophil and macrophages proteases, but proteases from other cells such as lung fibroblasts, and myofibroblasts, and dendritic cells may also be involved.

3.4 Role of the macrophage protease inhibitors TIMPs and cystatin C, and other protease inhibitors in emphysema

It is likely that it is the balance between macrophage proteases and their respective antiproteases that has a pathogenic role in emphysema. TIMPs are the endogenous inhibitors of MMPs; human AM release TIMP1 and TIMP2 (Shapiro et.,1992). AM from COPD patients release less TIMP1 *in vitro* than those from smokers without COPD and non-smokers (Pons et al., 2005), predisposing to proteolysis by MMPs. TIMP3 is the only TIMP that binds strongly to the extracellular matrix. TIMP3 knockout mice demonstrate progressive airspace enlargement and enhanced collagen degradation without inflammation or increased elastin breakdown (Leco et al., 2001). However, there are no reported associations between TIMP 3 polymorphisms and COPD. A polymorphism in the TIMP2 gene (G853A) was associated with COPD in a Japanese study (Hirano et al., 2001), and in an Egyptian population (Hegab et al., 2005).

Cystatin C is present in most biological fluids, and is a potent inhibitor of cathepsins. Cystatin C is a major product of AM (Chapman et al., 1990) and is secreted by AM from smokers at higher levels than non-smokers (Warfel et al., 1991) The concentrations of cathepsin L and its inhibitor cystatin C were both significantly increased in BAL fluid from smokers with emphysema compared with those without emphysema; however there was no significant difference in cathepsin L activity in BAL between the two groups (Takeyabu et al., 1998). There are no reports of deficiency or polymorphisms in cystatin C in relation to emphysema or COPD.

Polymorphisms in the Serpina2 gene, which encodes the protease nexin1 (plasminogen activator inhibitor type 1), were associated with COPD in a Boston population study (Demeo et al., 2006), and validated in two large family-based and case-control association studies (Zhu et al., 2007). Polymorphism of the SERPINA2 gene was also recently found associated with emphysema in consecutive autopsy cases in Japan (Fujimoto et al., 2010). Decreased activity of the plasminogen activator inhibitor type 1 in the lung can lead to increased activity of plasminogen , which can promote lung matrix degradation (Chapman et al.,1984).

3.5 Role of oxidants in protease-antiprotease imbalance

As indicated in a previously quoted review article on pathogenesis of COPD (MacNee, a2005), oxidants have a significant pathogenic role in COPD. The gaseous phase of cigarette smoke contains many reactive oxidants such as superoxide anion, nitric oxides and peroxynitrites, as reviewed recently (MacNee b2005; Lin & Thomas 2010). Oxidants and free radicals inhaled in tobacco smoke, can damage airway epithelial cells, and impair antioxidants, such as glutathione to non-reducible glutathione-aldehyde derivatives (van Der Toorn et al., 2007). Oxidants from tobacco smoke may also inactivate antiproteases, predisposing to a protease-antiprotease imbalance from the increased numbers of neutrophils and macrophages in smokers' lungs. Oxidants from cigarette smoke may also directly damage components of the lung connective tissure matrix, and interfere with elasin repair and synthesis (MacNee & Tuder 2009). Neutrophils and macrophages themselves when activated also release oxidants, such superoxides,, and nitric oxides, and contribute to the oxidative burden. Although antioxidants such as glutathione, catalase and superoxide dismutase protect the tissues against oxidants, the oxidant/antioxidant balance may tip in favor of oxidants leading to oxidative stress.

Patients with COPD have increased levels of hydrogen peroxide and of 8-isoprostane (a peroxidation product of arachidonic acid) in exhaled breath condensates compared with controls (MacNee b2005). Healthy smokers had reduced histone deacetylase activity in bronchial biopsies and in alveolar macrophages obtained by lavage, when compared with age matched nonsmoking controls (Ito, K., et al., 2001). These investigators also demonstrated that smoking resulted in a greater release of TNF-α from the alveolar macrophages when stimulated by IL-1β, which they considered was due to the suppressive effect of smoking on histone deacetylation. This suppressive effect on histone deacetylation results in increased acetylation, causes local unwinding of DNA, and allows increased inflammatory gene expression, which may contribute to the development of COPD. A later study confirmed decreased histone deacetylase acidity in resected lungs of COPD patients, and concluded that there was a progressive decrease in activity with increasing severity of COPD (Ito, K., et al., 2005). They also reported increased expression of IL-8 mRNA in lung tissue in COPD.

Oxidative stress may be determined non-invasively by measurement of oxidation products in exhaled breath condensates. According to a recent review article, the following markers of oxidative stress have been increased in exhaled breath condensates of subjects with COPD: hydrogen peroxide, nitrite, nitrosothiols, 8-isoprostane, and thiobarbituric acid reactive substances (Lee & Thomas, 2009). Oxidative stress is also indicated by the presence of biomarkers in blood indicative of lipid peroxidation., such as 4-hydroxy-2-nonenal (MacNee & Tuder 2009; Fischer, B.M., et al., 2011). The latter recent review article (Fischer, B.M., et al., 2011) also quoted published reports of increased levels of 4-hydroxy-2-nonenal, in both airways and alveoli of COPD patients, and also increased blood levels of malondialdehyde (an end product of lipid peroxidation) in COPD due to tobacco smoking as well as wood smoke exposure. 4-hydroxy-2-nonenal can increase gene expression of pro-inflammatory mediators such as IL-8, monocyte chemoattractant protein-1 (MacNee & Tuder 2009). Reactive oxygen species can also directly or indirectly induce pro-inflammatory mediators such as IL-1, TNF-α, Il-6, and IL-8 (Rahman & Adcock 2006).

The mRNA of inflammatory cytokines, chemokines, oxidant and antioxidant enzymes, proteases and antiproteases was evaluated in peripheral lung tissues from 14 COPD subjects and compared with 19 subjects without COPD undergoing lung resection for lung cancer (Tomaki, M., et al., 2007). They reported that mRNA, for catalase, two glutathion S-transferases, microsomal epoxide hydrolase, and TIMP2 were significantly decreased in COPD lung tissues compared with the non-COPD controls. On the other hand, the expressions of mRNA for IL-1β, IL-8, and monocyte chemotactic protein-1 (MCP-1) were significantly increased in COPD lungs. Most of these changes were also associated with cigarette smoking. Their data suggest that in addition to the impairment in antioxidant defenses, upregulation of cytokines and chemokines may be involved the development of COPD.

3.6 Role of inflammatory mediators and cytokines in protease-antiprotease imbalance

The last paragraph of page 4, reviewed the effects of TNF-α and IL-1β, on inducing expression of MMP9 by human macrophages without increasing its inhibitor TIMP1, predisposing to possible protease-antiprotease imbalance. In this section, I will briefly discuss these 2 pro-inflammatory cytokines and an additional one IL-8, which have been included in a review article on inflammatory mediators (Chung, K.F., 2005).

Imbalances between IL-1β and its antagonists in COPD have been reported in 15 patients with stable COPD compared with age matched healthy controls (Sapey, E., et al., 2009). Although mean concentrations of IL-1β in COPD were not different from controls, mean concentrations of their receptor antagonists (IL-RA & IL-1sRII) were markedly reduced, suggesting that IL-1β may have pathogenic role in COPD. In contrast, there were no difference in TNF-α and its antagonists in COPD patients compared with controls. A case control trial in Egyptian subjects over 60 years compared 3 groups of 30 subjects matched by age and sex, consisting of healthy subjects, COPD without any comorbidities, and COPD with cardiovascular disease but no other comorbidities (Amer, M.S., et al., 2010). There was no significant difference in the serum levels of IL-1β, TNF-α, or C reactive protein (CRP) between the control subjects and the COPD subjects with no cardiac disease. The group with cardiovascular disease had increased IL-1β and CRP (but not TNF-α) levels compared with the other 2 groups. However, the increase in IL-1β and CRP cannot be definitely attributed to the more severe COPD in the 3rd group, since it could be secondary to the cardiovascular comorbidity.

A study from Korea evaluated four potentially functional polymorphisms in the IL-1β in 311 COPD patients and 386 healthy controls and found polymorphisms that significantly increased the odds ratio of developing COPD (Lee, J.M., et al., 2008). In addition, they reported that a polymorphism in the Il-1β receptor antagonist gene IL-1RN afforded some protection.

Induced sputum from patients with moderate to severe COPD, had increased neutrophils, and increased levels of IL-8 and TNF-α, when compared with that of healthy cigarette smokers and normal non-smoking controls, (Keatings, V.M., et al., 1996). The increase in IL-8 was confirmed in a later study evaluating IL-8 in bronchoalveolar lavage fluid of COPD patients compared with controls (Pesci, A., et al., 1998).

Cytokine mRNA for IL-8, macrophage inflammatory protein-1α (MIP-1α), and MCP-1 were quantified using laser-capture microdissection of human bronchial epithelial cells and alveolar macrophages (Fuke, S., et al., 2004). The authors found that mRNA levels for IL-8, MIP-1α and MCP-1 were higher in bronchial epithelial cells of smokers with airflow obstruction and/or emphysema, compared with results in smokers without airflow obstruction or emphysema. However, there was no difference in macrophage mRNA levels for these cytokines between the 2 groups. Their findings support the role of the bronchiolar cells as the source of these increased chemokine levels in early COPD.

Although TNF-α has a major pathogenic role in experimental emphysema (Churg, A., et al., 2004), it does not appear to be as implicated in emphysema in human COPD. One study compared gene polymorphism in 169 Dutch COPD patients compared with Dutch controls, and reported an increased frequency of the G/A genotype in patients without radiological emphysema (Kucukaycan, M., et al., 2002). Another study from Italy compared 63 male patients with COPD with 86 healthy controls, and found no difference in gene polymorphisms between the two groups (Ferrarotti, I., et al., 2003).

It is likely that the pathogenic role of mediators and cytokines will be elucidated in multicenter studies evaluating pathogenetic mechanisms in COPD in association with large longitudonal clinical trials.

3.7 Role of T-lymphocytes and cell mediated immunity

Smokers with symptoms of chronic bronchitis and airflow limitation undergoing lung resection for a localized lesion were found to have increased numbers of CD8+ T-lymphocytes infiltrating the airway wall, which were increased compared with smokers with normal lung function, while the number of neutrophils, macrophages, and CD4+ T-lymphocytes were similar in the two groups (Saetta, M., et al., 1998). This suggested a pathogenic role for CD8+ lymphocytes in the development and progression of COPD. The subject of the role of lymphocytes in COPD is well covered by a recent review article (Gadgil & Duncan 2008). T lymphocytes can cause tissue injury either directly by cytolysis or by secreting pro-inflammatory mediators. Moreover, peripheral T-cells , specially CD8+ cells are activated and secrete mediators (Gadjil, A., et al., 2006). CD8+ lymphocytes appear to have a role in the development and progression of COPD, as quoted from several references in the review (Gadgil & Duncan 2008). CD8+ T-lymphocytes can mediate cell death directly through secretion of cytotoxins such as granzyme and perforins, as quoted from other references (Gadgil & Duncan 2008).

CD4+ T-cells can initiate downstream immune processes by releasing activating cytokines, can amplify inflammatory reactions by other immune cells, and are essential for full adaptive immune cytotoxicity by lowering the threshold of activation and promoting survival of CD8+ T-cells (Gadgil & Duncan 2008). In addition, CD4+ T-cells are important for the activation of antibody producing B-cells. In a previous study, they reported finding circulating IgG autoantibodies against epithelial cells in about 70% of their COPD patients, as compared with 10% of non-smoking controls, and 13% of cigarette smokers without evidence of lung disease (Feghali-Bostwick, C.A., et al., 2008). There was also immune complex deposition in six end stage explanted lungs. These autoantibodies may have a pathogenic role in airway epithelial injury in COPD. Also, a number of studies indicate that the lymphocyte proliferations in COPD are driven by peptide antigens, and consider various possibilities such as microbial peptide antigens, adenoviral antigens, tobacco smoke related peptides, elastin peptides, and auto-antigens from apoptotic cells and cellular debris (Gadgil & Duncan 2008).

4. Apoptosis and emphysema

This is an exciting new area of intense investigation which will further elucidate pathogenetic mechanisms in emphysema and is likely to lead to specific therapies in the future. Apoptosis refers to programmed cell death, affecting the endothelial capillaries and the alveolar epithelium leading to the development of emphysema. This area of investigation was initiated by the landmark study reporting that chronic blockade of Vascular Endothelial Growth Factor (VEGEF) receptors in rats by a chemical SU5416, induced alveolar septal apoptosis and enlargement of the air spaces indicating emphysema (Kasahara et al., 2000). The apoptosis was mediated by caspase 3, a proteolytic enzyme inducing apoptosis, and was prevented by treatment with a caspase inhibitor. The topic of apoptosis is covered by recent reviews (Demedts et al., 2006; Tuder et al., 2006, Morissette et al., 2009, Macnee & Tuder 2009). Additionally, specific sections about alveolar cell apoptosis and proliferation, aging and senescence, as well as mediators and signaling pathways, are also covered in a comprehensive review article about the pathobiology of cigarette smoke-induced COPD (Yoshida & Tuder, 2008). The pathways in apoptosis are involved, but may be simplified to an extrinsic and intrinsic pathway, The extrinsic pathway is activated by extracellular death ligands, such as those related to TNF-α which result in activation of caspases (proteolytic enzymes involved in apoptosis). The intrinsic pathway is triggered by cellular or DNA injury leading to the release of cytochrome C and apoptosis.

4.1 Human studies

Investigators studying human lung specimens to evaluate MMPs by immunohistochemistry in lungs with emphysema compared with controls, also evaluated apoptosis by terminal deoxynucleotide transferase-mediated dUTP nick-end labeling (TUNEL) assays, and were the first to report increased endothelial cell apoptosis and, to a lesser extent alveolar epithelial apoptosis in emphysema (Segura-Valdez et al., 2000). In 2001, the investigators who showed that VEGEF blockade in rats induced apoptosis , reported results from human lungs (Kasahara et al., 2001). The number of apoptotic epithelial and endothelial cells in alveolar septa of emphysema lungs per unit of lung tissue nucleic acid was about double in emphysema compared with normal lungs. In addition, VEGF, its receptor protein and mRNA expression were reduced in emphysema lungs, suggesting that apoptosis due to a decrease in endothelial maintenance factors may have a pathogenic role in emphysema, However another study reported no significant difference in apoptotic index in the lungs of 10 smokers with emphysema compared with 5 smokers without emphysema (Majo et a. 2001). Another group reported increased apoptosis of alveolar epithelial and endothelial cells as well as mesenchymal cells in lung tissue from 10 emphysema patients, compared with 6 controls without emphysema (Imai et al.,2005), and there was significant inverse correlation of apoptosis with lung surface area. They also evaluated cell proliferation by immunostaining for proliferating cell nuclear antigen (PCNA)., and reported that it was increased but was not correlated with apoptosis index or lung surface area. Other investigators evaluated apoptosis by flow cytometry in cells obtained by bronchoalveolar lavage in subjects with COPD, and compared results in 16 exsmokers with 13 current smokers, and 20 non-smoking volunteers (Hodge et al., 2005). There was a mean 87% increase in apoptotic airway epithelial cells in COPD subjects, and a mean doubling of apoptosis by airway T lymphocytes compared with non-smoking volunteers, but there was no difference between COPD subjects still smoking and those who had quit. They concluded that this increased airway cell apoptosis in COPD persists despite smoking cessation.

A study from Japan sought to evaluate the turnover of alveolar wall cells in emphysema by comparing lung tissue specimens from 13 patients with emphysema who had lung volume reduction surgery, 7 asymptomatic smokers and 9 non-smokers undergoing lung resection for solitary lung cancers (Yokohori et., 2004). They reported that the percentages of alveolar wall cells undergoing apoptosis and proliferation were higher in the emphysema patients than asymptomatic smokers or non-smokers. They concluded that emphysema is a dynamic process in which both alveolar cell wall apoptosis and proliferation are recurring. The same investigators also demonstrated that activated caspase 3 (an enzyme inducing apostosis) when instilled into the lungs of mice resulted in alveolar wall destruction and emphysema (Aoshiba et al., 2003). A study of 16 end-stage lungs from subjects undergoing lung transplantation for advanced emphysema (7 were due to AAT deficiency) were compared with 6 unused donor lungs (Calabrese et al., 2005). The apoptotic index was significantly increased in the emphysema lungs compared with controls, but the alveolar proliferation was similar in emphysema and control lungs. They concluded that there was a marked imbalance between alveolar apoptosis and alveolar proliferation in advanced emphysema.

In a study in patients undergoing lobectomy for lung cancer, there was increased apoptosis of alveolar walls by TUNEL assay and increased proliferation of alveolar cells in 10 subjects with emphysema, when compared with lungs from 10 asymptomatic smokers, and 10 nonsmokers (LIU et al. 2009). They also demonstrated increased apoptosis and decreased numbers of Type II epithelial cells in the lungs with emphysema.

As a result of previous studies showing increased apoptosis in human lungs with emphysema (Yokohori et al., 2004), and induction of apoptosis by caspase 3 in mice (Aoshiba et al., 2003), these investigators (Aoshiba & Nagai, 2009) proposed a senescence hypothesis as a pathogenic mechanism in emphysema. They speculated that cellular senescence was the cause of the insufficient cellular proliferation in emphysema, and found that senescence markers were increased in emphysema lungs. They considered that smoking and aging caused alveolar and airway cells to senesce , and senescence decreased tissue repair resulting in reduced cell numbers .

5. Conclusions

Protease-antiprotease imbalance is likely to have a major pathogenic role in the development of emphysema in severe AAT deficiency. However the case in non-AAT deficient smokers is not firmly established, but is supported by several studies showing associations of emphysema with proteolyic enzyme levels or message expression, and by the association of polymorphisms with decline in lung function. It is also supported by a review of animal models of cigarette smoke-induced COPD, where the opening sentence of the Abstract supports the protease-antiprotease hypothesis of emphysema (Churg, A., et al., 2008). However there are other mechanisms that play a pathogenic role such as oxidants, inflammation, and T lymphocyte induced immunity. Apoptosis is likely to have a significant pathogenic role in emphysema and may be amenable to therapy in the future.

6. Acknowledgements

I thank Andrew Sandford, Allison Wallace, Hong Li, Takeo Ishii, and Selvarani Vimanathalan for their collaboration in studies on alveolar macrophage proteases and antiproteases in relation to emphysema.

7. References

Abboud, R. , & Vimanalathan, S. (2008). Pathogenesis of COPD. Part I. The role of protease-antiprotease imbalance in emphysema. *Int J Tuberc Lung Dis,* Vol. 12, No. 4, (April 2008), pp. (361-367).

Abboud, R.T., Fera, T., Richter, A., Tabona, M.Z., & Johal, S. (1985). Acute effect of smoking on the functional activity of alpha1-protease inhibitor in bronchoalveolar lavage fluid. *Am Rev Respir Dis,* Vol. 131, No. 1, (January 1985), pp. (79-85)

Abboud, R.T., Fera, T., Johal, S., Richter, A., & Gibson, N. (1986). Effect of smoking on plasma neutrophil elastase levels. *J Lab Clin Med,* Vol. 108, No. 4, (October 1986), pp. (294-300)

Abboud, R.T., Ofulue, A.F., Sansores, R.H., & Muller, N.L. (1998). Relationship of alveolar macrophage plasminogen activator and elastase activities to lung function and CT evidence of emphysema. *Chest,* Vol. 113, No. 5, (May 1998), pp. (1257-1263)

Amer, M.S., Wahba, H.M., Ashmawi, S.S., et al., (2010). Proinflammatory cytokines in Egyptian elderly with chronic obstructive pulmonary disease. *Lung India,* Vol. 27, No.4, (October 2010), pp. (225-229)

Aoshiba, K., Yokohori, N., & Nagai, A. (2003). Alveolar wall apoptosis causes lung destruction and emphysematous changes. *Am J Respir Cell Mol Biol,* Vol. 28, No. 5, (May 2003), pp. 555-562)

Aoshiba, K., & Nagai A. (2009). Senescence hypothesis for the pathogenetic mechanism of chronic obstructive pulmonary disease. *Proc Am Thorac Soc,* Vol. 6, No. 7, (December 2009), pp. (596-601)

Atkinson, J.J., Lutey, B.A., & Suzuki, Y. et al., (2011). The role of matrix metalloproteinase-9 in cigarette smoke-induced emphysema. *Am J Respir Crit Care Med,* Vol. 183, No. 7, (April 2011), pp. (876-884)

Betsuyaku, T., Yoshioka, A., & Nishimura, M. et al., (1995). Neutrophil elastase associated with alveolar macrophages from older volunteers. *Am J Respir Crit Care Med,* Vol. 151, No. 2, (February 1995), pp. (436-442)

Boudier, C., Pelletier, A., Pauli, G., & Bieth, J.G. (1983). The functional activity of a1-proteinase inhibitor in bronchoalveolar lavage fluids from healthy human smokers and non-smokers. *Clin Chim Acta,* Vol. 132, No. 3, (August 1983), pp. (309-315)

Calabrese, F., Giacometti, C., & Beghe, B. et al., (2005). Marked alveolar apoptosis/proliferation imbalance in end-stage emphysema. *Respir Res,* Vol. 6, No. 14, (February 2005)

Campbell, E.J., White, R.R., Senior, R.M., Rodriguez, R.J., & Kuhn, C. (1979). Receptor-mediated binding and internalization of leukocyte elastase by alveolar macrophages in vitro. *J Clin Invest,* Vol. 64, No. 3, (September 1979), pp. 824-833)

Carp, H., Miller, F., Hoidal, J.R., & Janoff, A. (1982). Potential mechanism of emphysema: alpha 1-proteinase inhibitor recovered from lungs of cigarette smokers contains oxidized methionine and has decreased elastase inhibitory capacity. *Proc Natl Acad Sci USA,* Vol. 79, No. 6, (March 1982), pp. (2041-2045)

Chapman, H.A.Jr., Stone, O.L., & Vavrin, Z. (1984). Degradation of fibrin and elastin by intact human alveolar macrophages in vitro. Characterization of a plasminogen activator and its role in matrix degradation. *J Clin Invest,* Vol. 73, No. 3, (March 1984), pp. 806-815)

Chapman, H.A.Jr., & Stone, O.L. (1984). Comparison of live human neutrophil and alveolar macrophage elastolytic activity in vitro. Relative resistance of macrophage elastolytic activity to serum and alveolar proteinase inhibitors. *J Clin Invest,* Vol. 74, No. 5, (November 1984), pp. (1693-1700)

Chapman, H.A.Jr., Reilly, J.J.Jr., Yee, R., & Grubb, A. (1990). Identification of cystatin C, a cysteine proteinase inhibitor, as a major secretory product of human alveolar macrophages in vitro. *Am Rev Respir Dis,* Vol. 141, No. 3, (March 1990), pp. (698-705)

Chung, K.F. (2005). Inflammatory mediators in chronic obstructive pulmonary disease. *Curr Drug Targets Inflamm Allergy,* Vol. 4, No. 6, (December 2005), pp. (619-625)

Churg, A., Wang, R.D., & Tai, H. et al., (2003). Macrophage metalloelastase mediates acute cigarette smoke-induced inflammation via tumor necrosis factor-α release. *Am J Respir Crit Care Med,* Vol. 167, No. 8, (April 2003), pp. (1083-1089)

Churg, A., Wang, R.D., Tai, H., Wang, X., Xie, C., & Wright, J.L. (2004). Tumor necrosis factor-alpha drives 70% of cigarette smoke-induced emphysema in the mouse. *Am J Respir Crit Care Med,* Vol. 170, No. 5, (September 2004), pp. (492-498)

Churg, A., Cosio, M., & Wright, J.L. (2008). Mechanisms of cigarette smoke-induce COPD: insights from animal models. *Am J Physiol Lung Cell Mol Physiol,* Vol. 294, No. 4, (April 2008), pp. (L612-L631)

D'Armiento, J., Dalal, S.S., Okada, Y., Berg, R.A., & Chada, K. (1992). Collagenase expression in the lungs of transgenic mice causes pulmonary emphysema. *Cell,* Vol. 71, No. 6, (December 1992), pp. (955-961)

Demedts, I.K., Morel-Montero, A., Lebecque, S., Pacheco, Y., Cataldo, D., Joos, G.F., Pauwels, R.A., & Brusselle, G.G. (2006). Elevated MMP-12 protein levels in induced sputum from patients with COPD. *Thorax,* Vol. 61, No. 3, (Mar 2006), pp. (196–201)

Demedts, I.K., Demoor, T., & Bracke, K.R. et al., (2006). Role of apoptosis in the pathogenesis of COPD and pulmonary emphysema. *Respir Res,* Vol. 7, No. 53, (March 2006)

Demeo, D.L., Mariani, T.J., & Lange, C. et al., (2006). The Serpine2 gene is associated with chronic obstructive pulmonary disease . *Am J Hum Genetics,* Vol. 78, No. 2, (February 2006), pp. (253-264)

Feghali-Bostwick, C.A., Gadjil, A.S., Otterbein, L.E., et al., (2008). Autoantibodies in patients with chronic obstructive pulmonary disease. *Am J Respir Crit Care Med,* Vol. 177, No. 2, (January 2008), pp. (156-163)

Fera, T., Abboud, R.T., Richter, A., & Johal, S. (1986). Acute effect of smoking on elastase-like activity and immunologic neutrophil elastase levels in bronchoalveolar lavage. *Am Rev Respir Dis,* Vol. 133, Vol. 4, (April 1986), pp. (568-573)

Ferrarotti, I., Zorzetto, M., Beccaria, M., et al., (2003). Tumour necrosis factor family genes in a phenotype of COPD associated with emphysema. *Eur Respir J,* Vol. 21, No. 3, (March 2003), pp. (444-449)

Finkelstein, R., Fraser, R.S., Ghezzo, H., & Cosio, M.G. (1995). Alveolar inflammation and its relation to emphysema in smokers. *Am J Respir Crit Care Med,* Vol. 152, No. 5, (November 1995), pp. (1666-1672)

Finlay, G.A., O'Driscoll, L.R., & Russell, K.J. et al., (1997). Matrix metalloproteinase expression and production by alveolar macrophages in emphysema. *Am J Respir Crit Care Med,* Vol. 156, No. 1, (July 1997), pp. (240-247)

Fischer, B.M., Pavlisko, E., Voynow, J.A. (2011). Pathogenic Triad in COPD: oxidative stress, protease-antiprotease imbalance, and inflammation. *Int J Chron Obstruct Pulmon Dis,* Vol. 6, (August 2011), pp. (413-421)

Foronjy, R.F., Okada, Y., Cole, R., & D'Armiento, J. (2003). Progressive adult-onset emphysema in transgenic mice expressing human MMP-1 in the lung. *Am J Physiol Lung Cell Mol Physiol,* Vol. 284, No. 5, (May 2003), pp. (L727-737)

Fujimoto, K., Ikeda, S., & Arai, T. et al., (2010). Polymorphism of Serpina 2 gene is associated with pulmonary emphysema in consecutive autopsy cases. *BMC Med Genet,* Nov; 11, 159, (November 2010)

Fujita, J., Nelson, N.L., & Daughton, D.M. et al., (1990). Evaluation of elastase and antielastase balance in patients with chronic bronchitis and pulmonary emphysema. *Am Rev Respir Dis,* Vol. 142, No. 1, (July 1990), pp. 57-62)

Fuke, S., Betsuyaku, T., Nasuhara, Y., et al., (2004). Chemokines in bronchiolar epithelium in the development of chronic obstructive pulmonary disease. *Am J Respir Cell Mol Biol,* Vol. 31, No. 4, (June 2004), pp. (405-412)

Gadek, J.E., Fells, G.A,. & Crystal, R.G. (1979). Cigarette smoking induces functional antiprotease deficiency in the lower respiratory tract of humans. *Science,* Vol. 206, No. 4424, (December 1979), pp. (1315-1316)

Gadgil, A., & Duncan, S.R. (2008).Role of T-lymphocytes and pro-inflammatory mediators in the pathogenesis of chronic obstructive pulmonary disease. *Int J Chron Obstruct Pulmon Dis,* Vol. 3, No. 4, (2008), pp. (531-541)

Gadgil, A., Zhu, X., Sciurba, F.C., Duncan, S.R. (2006). Altered T-cell phenotypes in chronic obstructive pulmonary disease. *Proc Am Thorac Soc,* Vol. 3, No. 6. (August 2006) pp. (487-488)

Golovatch, P., Mercer, B.A., Lemaitre, V. et al., (2009). Role for cathepsin K in emphysema in smoke exposed guinea pigs. *Exp Lung Res,* Vol. 38, No. 8, (October 2009), pp. (631-645)

Gross, P., Pfitzer, E.A., Toker, A. et al., (1965). Experimental emphysema: its production with papain in normal and silicotic rats. *Arch Environ Health,* Vol. 11, (July 1965), pp. (50-58)

Haq, I., Chappell, S., Johnson, S.R. et al., (2010). Association of MMP-12 polymorphisms with severe and very severe COPD: a case control study of MMPs-1, 9 and 12 in a European population. *BMC Med Genet,* Jan 15; 11: 7, (January 2010)

Hautamaki, R.D., Kobayashi, D.K., Senior, R.M., & Shapiro, S.D. (1997). Requirement for macrophage elastase for cigarette smoke-induced emphysema in mice. *Science,* Vol. 277, No. 5334, (September 1997), pp. (2002-2004)

Hegab, A.E., Sakamoto, T., Uchida, Y. et al., (2005). Association analysis of tissue inhibitor of metalloproteinase2 gene polymorphisms with COPD in Egyptians. *Respir Med,* Vol. 99, No. 1, (January 2005), pp. (107-110)

Hirano, K., Sakamoto, T., Uchida, Y. et al., (2001). Tissue inhibitor of metalloproteinases-2 gene polymorphisms in chronic obstructive pulmonary disease. *Eur Respir J,* Vol. 18, No. 5, (November 2001), pp. (748-52)

Hodge, S., Hodge, G., Holmes, M., & Reynolds, P.M. (2005). Increased airway epithelial and T-cell apoptosis in COPD remains despite smoking cessation. *Eur Respir J,* Vol. 25, No. 3, (March 2005), pp. (447-454)

Imai, K., Dalal, S.S., Chen, E.S. et al., (2001). Human collagenase (matrix metalloproteinase-1) expression in the lungs of patients with emphysema. *Am J Respir Crit Care Med,* Vol. 163, No. 3, (March 2001), pp. (786-791)

Imai, K., Mercer, B.A., & Schulman, L.L. et al., (2005). Correlation of lung surface area to apoptosis and proliferation in human emphysema. *Eur Respir J,* Vol. 25, No. 2, (February 2005), pp. (250-258)

Ito, I., Nagai, S., & Handa, T. et al., (2005). Matrix Metalloproteinase-9 Promoter Polymorphism Associated with Upper Lung Dominant Emphysema. *Am J Respir Crit Care Med,* Vol. 172, No. 11, (December 2005), pp. (1378-1382)

Ito, K., Lim, S., Caramori, K.F., et al., (2001). Cigarette smoking reduces histone deacetylase 2 expression, enhances cytokine expression, and inhibits glucocorticoid actions in alveolar macrophages. *FASEB J,* Vol. 15, (February 5, 2001), Published on line

Ito, K., Ito, M., Elliot, W.M., et al., (2005). Decreased histone deacetylase activity in chronic obstructive pulmonary disease. *N Engl J Med,* Vol. 352, No. 19, (May 2005) pp. (1967-1976)

Janoff, A., Sloan, B., & Weinbaum, G. et al., (1977). Experimental emphysema induced with purified human neutrophil elastase: tissue localization of the instilled protease. *Am Rev Respir Dis,* Vol. 115, No. 3, (March 1977), pp. (461-478)

Janoff A. (1985). Elastases and emphysema. Current assessment of the protease-antiprotease hypothesis. *Am Rev Respir Dis,* Vol. 132 No. 2, (August 1985), pp. (417-433)

Kasahara, Y., Tuder, R.M., & Taraseeviciene-Stewart, L. et al., (2000). Inhibition of VEGF receptors causes lung cell apoptosis and emphysema. *J Clin Invest,* Vol. 106, No. 11, (December 2000), pp. (1311-1319)

Kasahara, Y., Tuder, R.M., & Vool, C.D. et al., (2001). Endothelial cell death and decreased expression of of vascular endothelial growth factor receptor 2 in emphysema. *Am J Respir Crit Care Med,* Vol. 163, No. 3, (March 2001), pp. (737-744)

Kidokoro, Y., Kravis, T.C., Moser, K.M., Taylor, J.C., & Crawford, I.P. (1977). Relationship of leukocyte elastase concentration to severity of emphysema in homozygous alpha1-antitrypsin-deficient persons. *Am Rev Respir Dis,* Vol. 115, No. 5, (May 1977), pp. (793-803)

Korytina, G.F., Akhmadishina, L.Z., Ianbaeva, D.G. et al., (2008). Polymorphism in promoter regions of matrix metalloproteinases (MMP1, MMP9, and MMP12) in chronic obstructive pulmonary disease patients [Russian, English Abstract]. *Genetika,* Vol. 44, No. 2, (February 2008), pp. 242-249)

Kucukayan, M., Van Kugten, M., Pennings, H.J., et al., (2002). Tumor necrosis factor-alpha +489G/A gene polymorphisms is associated with chronic obstructive pulmonary disease. *Respir Res,* 2002; 3:29. Epub 2002, November 29

Laurell, C.B., & Eriksson, S. (1963). The electrophoretic alpha-1-globulin pattern of serum in α1-antitrypsin deficiency. *Scand J Clin Invest,* Vol. 15, (1963), pp. (132-140)

Leco, K.J., Waterhouse, P., Sanchez, O.H. et al., (2001). Spontaneous air space enlargement in the lungs of mice lacking tissue inhibitor of metalloproteinases-3 (TIMP-3). *J Clin Invest,* Vol. 108, No. 6, (September 2001), pp. (817-829)

Lee, J.M., Kang, Y.R., Park, S.H., et al., (2008). Polymorphisms in interleukin-1β and its receptor antagonist genes and the risk of chronic obstructive pulmonary disease in a Korean population: a case control study. *Respir Med*, Vol. 102, No. 9, (September 2008), pp. (1311-1320)

Lee, W., & Thomas, P.S. (2009). Oxidative stress in COPD and its measurement through exhaled breath condensate. *Clin Transl Sci*, Vol. 2, No. 2, (April 2009), pp. (150-155)

Lin, J-L., & Thomas, P.S. (2010). Current perspectives of oxidative stress and its measurement in chronic obstructive pulmonary disease. *COPD:* Vol. 7, No. 4, (August 2010), pp. (291-306)

Liu, H., Ma, L., Wu, J., Wang, K., & Chen, X.J. (2009). Apoptosis of alveolar wall cells in chronic obstructive pulmonary disease patients with pulmonary emphysema is involved in emphysematous changes. *Huazhong Univ Sci Technolog Med Sci*, Vol. 29, No. 4, (August 2009), pp. (466-469)

MacNee, W. (a2005). Pathogenesis of Chronic Obstructive Pulmonary Disease. *Proc Am Thoracic Soc*, Vol. 2, No. 4, (2005), pp. (258-266)

MacNee, W. (b2005). Pulmonary and systemic oxidant/antioxidant imbalance in chronic obstructive pulmonary disease. Proc Am Thoracic Soc, Vol. 2, No. 1, (January 2005), pp. (50-60)

MacNee, W., & Tuder, R.M. (2009). New paradigms in the pathogenesis of COPD I. *Proc Am Thoracic Soc*, Vol. 6, No. 6, (September 2009), pp. (527-531)

Majo, J., Ghezzo, H., & Cosio, M.G. (2001). Lymphocyte population and apoptosis in the lungs of smokers and their relation to emphysema. *Eur Respir J*, Vol. 17, No. 5, (May 2001), pp. (946-953), ISSN 0903-1936

Minematsu, N., Nakamura, H., Tateno, H., Nakajima, T., & Yamaguchi, K. (2001). Genetic polymorphism in matrix metalloproteinase-9 and pulmonary emphysema. *Biochem Biophys Res Commun*, Vol. 289, No. 1, (November 2001), pp. (116-119)

Molet, S., Belleguic, C., & Lena, H. et al., (2005). Increase in macrophage elastase (MMP-12) in lungs from patients with chronic obstructive pulmonary disease. *Inflamm Res*, Vol. 54, No. 1, (January 2005), pp. 31-36)

Morissette, M.C., Parent, J., & Milot, J. (2009). Alveolar epithelial and endothelial cell apoptosis in emphysema: what we know and what we need to know. *Int J Chron Obstruct Pulmon Dis*, Vol. 4, (April 2009), pp. (19-31)

Morrison, H.M., Welgus, H.G., Stockley, R.A., Burnett, D., & Campbell, E.J. (1990). Inhibition of human leucocyte elastase bound to elastin: relative ineffectiveness and two mechanisms of inhibitory activity. *Am J Respir Cell Mol Biol*, Vol. 2, No. 3, (March 1990), pp. (263-269)

Muley, T., Wiebel, M., Schulz, V., & Ebert, W. (1994). Elastinolytic activity of alveolar macrophages in smoking-associated pulmonary emphysema. *Clin Investig*, Vol. 72, No. 4, (March 1994), pp. (269-276)

Niewoehner, D.E., Kleinerman, J., & Rice, D.B. (1974). Pathologic changes in the peripheral airways of young cigarette smokers. *N Engl J Med*, Vol. 291, No. 15, (October 1974), pp. (755-758)

Ohnishi, K., Takagi, M., Kurokawa, Y., Satomi, S., & Konttinen, Y.T. (1998). Matrix metalloproteinase-mediated extracellular matrix protein degradation in human pulmonary emphysema. *Lab Invest*, Vol. 78, No. 9, (September 1998), pp. (1077-1087)

Omachi, T.A., Eisner, M.D., & Rames, A. et al., (2011). Matrix metalloproteinase-9 predicts pulmonary status declines in α1-antitrypsin deficiency. *Respir Res*, Vol. 12, No. 35, (March 2011)

Park, J.W., Ryter, S.W., & Choi, A.M. (2007). Functional significance of apoptosis in chronic obstructive pulmonary disease. *COPD*, Vol. 4, No. 4, (December 2007), pp. (347-353)

Pons, A.R., Sauleda, J., & Noguera, A. et al., (2005). Decreased macrophage release of TGF-beta and TIMP-1 in chronic obstructive pulmonary disease. *Eur Respir J*, Vol. 26, No. 1, (July 2005), pp. (60-66)

Rahman, I., & Adcock, I.M. (2006). Oxidative stress and redox regulation of lung inflammation in COPD. Eur Respir J, Vol. 28, No. 1, (July 2006), pp. (219-242)

Reilly, J.J., Mason, R.W., & Chen, P. et al., (1989). Synthesis and processing of cathepsin L, an elastase, by human alveolar macrophages. *Biochem J*, Vol. 257, No. 2, (January 1989), pp. 493-498)

Reilly, J.J., Chen, P., & Sailor, L.Z. et al., (1991). Cigarette smoking induces an elastolytic cysteine proteinase in macrophages distinct from cathepsin L. *Am J Physiol*, Vol. 261, No. 2, (August 1991), pp. (L41-48)

Russell, R.E., Culpitt, S.V., & DeMatos, C. et al., (2002). Release and activity of` matrix metalloproteinase-9 and tissue inhibitor of metalloproteinase-1 by alveolar macrophages from patients with chronic obstructive pulmonary disease. *Am J Respir Cell Mol Biol*, Vol. 26, No. 5, (May 2002), pp. (602-609)

Russell, R.E., Thorley, A., & Murray, R. et al., (2002). Alveolar macrophage-mediated elastolysis: roles of matrix metalloproteinases, cysteine, and serine proteases. *Am J Physiol Lung Cell Mol Physiol*, Vol. 283, No. 4, (October 2002), pp. (L867-L873)

Saren, P., Welgus, H.G., & Kovanen, P.T. (1996). TNF-alpha and IL-1beta selectively induce expression of 92-kDa gelatinase by human macrophages. *J Immunol*, Vol. 157, No. 9, (November 1996), pp. (4159-4165)

Sapey, E. Ahmad, A., Bayley, D., et al., (2009).Imbalances between interleukin-1 and tumor necrosis factor agonists and antagonists in stable COPD. *J Clin Immunol*, Vol. 29, No.4, (July 2009), pp. (508-516)

Segura-Valdez, L., Pardo, A., & Gaxiola, M. et al., (2000). Upregulation of gelatinases A and B, collagenases 1 and 2, and increased parenchymal cell death in COPD. *Chest*, Vol. 117, No. 3, (March 2000), pp. (684-694)

Senior, R.M., Tegner, H., & Kuhn, C. et al., (1977). The induction of pulmonary emphysema with leukocyte elastase. *Am Rev Respir Dis*, Vol. 116, No. 3, (September 1977), pp. (469-475)

Senior, R.M., Griffin, G.L., & Fliszar, C.J. et al., (1991). Human 92- and 72-kilodalton type IV collagenases are elastases. *J Biol Chem*, Vol. 266, No. 12, (April 1991), pp. (7870-7875)

Shapiro, S.D., Kobayashi, D.K., & Welgus, H.G. (1992). Identification of TIMP-2 in human alveolar macrophages. Regulation of biosynthesis is opposite to that of metalloproteinases and TIMP-1. *J Biol Chem*, Vol. 267, No. 20, (July 1992), pp. (13890-13894)

Shapiro, S.D., Kobayashi, D., Pentland, A.P., & Welgus, H.G. (1993). Induction of macrophage metalloproteinases by extracellular matrix. Evidence for enzyme- and substrate-specific responses involving prostaglandin-dependent mechanisms. *J Biol Chem*, Vol. 268, No. 11, (April 1993), pp. (8170-8175)

Shapiro, S.D., Kobayashi, D.K., & Ley, T.J. (1993). Cloning and characterization of a unique elastolytic metalloproteinase produced by human alveolar macrophages. *J Biol Chem*, Vol. 268, No. 32, (November 1993), pp. (23824-23829)

Shapiro, S.D., Goldstein, N.M., & Houghton, A.M. et al., (2003). Neutrophil elastase contributes to cigarette smoke-induced emphysema in mice. *Am J Pathol*, Vol. 163, No. 6, (December 2003), pp. (2329-2335)

Shi, G.P., Munger, J.S., Meara, J.P., Rich, D.H., & Chapman, H.A. (1992). Molecular cloning and expression of human alveolar macrophage cathepsin S, an elastinolytic cysteine protease. *J Biol Chem,* Vol. 267, No. 11, (April 1992), pp. (7258-7262)

Shiomi, T., Okada, Y., & Foronjy, R. et al., (2003). Emphysematous changes are caused by degradation of type III collagen in transgenic mice expressing MMP-1. *Exp Lung Res,* Vol. 29, No. 1, (Jan-Feb 2003), pp. (1-15)

Stone, P.J., Calore, J.D., McGowan, S.E., Bernardo, J., Snider, G.L., & Franzblau, C. (1983). Functional a1-protease inhibitor in the lower respiratory tract of cigarette smokers is not decreased. *Science,* Vol. 221, No. 4616, (September 1983), pp. (1187-1189)

Takahashi, H., Ishidoh, K., & Muno, D. et al., (1993). Cathepsin L activity is increased in alveolar macrophages and bronchoalveolar lavage fluid of smokers. *Am Rev Respir Dis,* Vol. 147, No. 6, (June 1993), pp. (1562-1568)

Takeyabu, K., Betsuyaku, T., & Nishimura, M. et al., (1998). Cysteine proteinases and cystatin C in bronchoalveolar lavage fluid from subjects with subclinical emphysema. *Eur Respir J,* Vol. 12, No. 5, (November 1998), pp. (1033-1039)

Tomaki, M., Sugiura, H., Koarai A., et al., (2007). Decreased expression of antioxidant enzymes and increased expression of chemokines in COPD lung. *Pulm Pharmacol Ther,* Vol.20, No. 5, (July 2007), pp. (596-605)

Tuder, R.M., Yoshida, T., Arap, W., Pasqualini, R., & Petrache, I. (2006). State of the art. Cellular and molecular mechanisms of alveolar destruction in emphysema: an evolutionary perspective. *Proc Am Thorac Soc,* Vol. 3, No. 6, (August 2006), pp. (503-510)

Van der Toorn, M., Smit-de Vries, M.P., Slebos, D.J., et al., (2007). Cigarette smoke irreversibly modifies glutathione in airway epithelial cells. *Am J Physiol Lung Cell Mol Physiol,* Vol.293, No. 5, (November 2007), pp. (L1156-1162)

Wallace, A.M., Sandford, A.J., & English, J.C., et al., (2008). Matrix metalloproteinase expression by human alveolar macrophages in relation to emphysema. *COPD,* Vol. 5, No. 1, (February 2008), pp. (13-23)

Warfel, A.H., Cardozo, C., Yoo, O.H., & Zucker-Franklin D. (1991). Cystatin C and cathepsin B production by alveolar macrophages from smokers and nonsmokers. *J Leukoc Biol,* Vol. 49, No. 1, (January 1991), pp. (41-47)

Yokohori, N., Aoshiba, K., & Nagai, A. (2004). Increased levels of cell death and proliferation in alveolar wall cells in patients with pulmonary emphysema. *Chest,* Vol. 125, No. 2 (February 2004), pp. (626-632)

Yoshida, T., & Tuder, R.M. (2007). Pathobiology of cigarette smoke-induced chronic obstructive pulmonary disease. *Physiol Rev,* Vol. 87, No. 3, (July 2007), pp. (1047-1082)

Zhou, M., Huang, S.G., & Wan, H.Y. et al., (2004). Genetic polymorphism in matrix metalloproteinase-9 and the susceptibility to chronic obstructive pulmonary disease in Han population of south China. *Chin Med J (Engl),* Vol. 117, No. 10, (October 2004), pp. (1481-1484)

Zhu, G., Warren, L., & Aponte, J. et al., (2007). The SERPINE2 gene is associated with chronic obstructive disease in two large populations. *Am J Respir Crit Care Med,* Vol. 176, No. 2, (July 2007), pp. (167-173)

2

Innate Immunity of Airway Epithelium and COPD

Shyamala Ganesan and Uma S. Sajjan
University of Michigan, USA

1. Introduction

The mammalian immune system consists of two branches- innate and adaptive immune systems and together they provide protection against infection. Innate immunity is a first line of host defense and is responsible for immediate recognition of pathogens to prevent microbial invasion. In addition innate immune responses also stimulate adaptive immune system (Medzhitov and Janeway, 1997). Cellular components of innate immune system include mucosal epithelial cells, macrophages, neutrophils, natural killer cells, basophils, eosinophils and others. The airway mucosa represents the body's largest mucosal surface and is the first point of contact for inhaled microorganisms, environmental pollutants, airborne allergens and cigarette smoke (Diamond et al., 2000). Airway mucosa provides protection against potentially hazardous inhaled factors by multiple mechanisms. For instance, mucus secreted by the airway epithelium covers the apical surface of airway epithelium and traps inhaled microorganisms, allergens and particulate material. The trapped material is then cleared by mucociliary escalator away from lungs and towards the pharynx. Tight junctions between the polarized airway epithelial cells restrict the paracellular movement of solutes and ions, and prevent pathogens from gaining access to the submucosal compartment. In addition to its role as a physical barrier between environmental factors and internal milieu, airway epithelial cells also play a critical role in bridging innate and adaptive immune defenses (Hammad and Lambrecht, 2011; Kato and Schleimer, 2007). Airway epithelial cells express number of innate immune receptors also known as pattern recognition molecules, which recognizes pathogen-associated molecular patterns (PAMPS) or danger-associated molecular patterns (DAMPS) to initiate appropriate innate defense mechanisms. This includes elaboration of antimicrobial molecules, pro-inflammatory cytokines and chemokines that recruits and activates other mucosal innate immune cells. The responses of activated innate immune cells lead to recruitment of immune cells into epithelium or airway lumen and initiate adaptive immune responses. Continuous exposure to environmental stimuli, such as cigarette smoke, noxious gases or other environmental hazards may lead to prolonged and aberrant activation of airway epithelial cells resulting in excessive expression of pro-inflammatory cytokines and chemokines that recruit large number of inflammatory cells into airway lumen. This in turn leads to persistent inflammation, airway damage and abnormal repair, impaired innate immune responses. There are reports suggesting that exposure to cigarette smoke also dampens the needed innate immune responses to infection, thereby promoting the persistence of infecting organism. This may result in delayed but sustained inflammation that can lead to progression of lung disease. In this chapter, we will discuss how the impaired innate immune defense mechanisms fail to provide protection against invading pathogens and its impact on progression of lung disease in patients with chronic obstructive pulmonary disease (COPD).

2. Barrier function of airway epithelium

Airway epithelium lines the entire airway mucosa. In normal adult human, the large airways are cartilaginous and mainly made up of ciliated cells, mucus producing goblet cells, undifferentiated columnar cells and basal cells with a capacity to multiply and differentiate into ciliated or goblet cells. Large airways are also surrounded by submucosal and serous glands. As the large airways branches out, it gradually becomes non-cartilaginous, loses surrounding submucosal and serous glands, the cells become more columnar and cuboidal, and Clara secreting cells replace goblet cells in the small airways. Airway epithelium also consists of other minor cell types such as neuroendocrine cells, dendritic cells and others.

The three essential components that contributes to barrier function of airway epithelium are mucociliary apparatus (Knowles and Boucher, 2002), intercellular tight and adherens junctions (Pohl et al., 2009) that regulates epithelial paracellular permeability, and secreted antimicrobial products that kill the inhaled pathogens (Bals and Hiemstra, 2004).

2.1 Mucociliary clearance

The primary players of mucociliary apparatus are mucus produced by goblet cells and submucosal glands that overlay the airway epithelium and cilia. Mucociliary dysfunction results in recurrent and persistent respiratory infections as evidenced in patients with cystic fibrosis, ciliary dyskinesia and COPD (Bhowmik et al., 2009; Jansen et al., 1995; Livraghi and Randell, 2007; Sethi, 2000). In COPD patients, the dysfunction of mucociliary clearance is due to combined effect of mucus hypersecretion, increased viscosity of mucus and dysfunction or loss of cilia (Mehta et al., 2008). The airway mucus is a viscoelastic gel and contains more than 200 proteins, and it is secreted by goblet cells that are present in the airway epithelium and by submucosal glands. The main components of airway mucus are mucins, which are high molecular weight glycoproteins and cross link to form structural framework of mucus barrier (Rose et al., 2001; Thornton et al., 2008). At least 12 mucins are detected in human lungs, of these MUC5AC and MUC5B are the predominant mucins in normal airways (Rose and Voynow, 2006). Airways infection with virus or bacteria, exposure to toxic agents such as cigarette smoke and pollutants that induce airway inflammation and oxidative stress have been shown to upregulate expression of MUC5AC and MUC5B (Borchers et al., 1999; Casalino-Matsuda et al., 2009; Dohrman et al., 1998; Gensch et al., 2004; Haswell et al., 2010; Shao et al., 2004). Cigarette smoke induces expression of number of inflammatory mediators including IL-1β, IL-8, TNF-α, MCP-1, leukotrienes through oxidative stress-related pathways from airway epithelial cells, resident macrophages and infiltrated neutrophils, which can increase mucus secretion (Adcock et al., 2011; Choi et al., 2010; Cohen et al., 2009; Mebratu et al., 2011). Cigarette smoke also causes mucus hypersecretion by increasing expression of hypoxia-induced factor 1 and growth factors such as TGF-β, and EGF ligands (Yu et al., 2011a, b). Smokers with COPD also show goblet cell metaplasia and submucosal gland hypertrophy (Innes et al., 2006). Increased EGF receptor expression and activation and increased expression of platelet activating factor caused by cigarette smoke are thought to play a role in development of goblet cell metaplasia (Curran and Cohn, 2010; Komori et al., 2001; O'Donnell et al., 2004). Cigarette smoke decreases water and ion transport by inhibiting apical chloride channel and basolaterally located potassium channel in primary human and mouse airway epithelial cells(Cohen et al., 2009; Savitski et al., 2009). This essentially reduces the periciliary liquid layer in which cilia can beat rapidly and also increases the viscosity of mucus resulting in reduced clearance of mucus from the airways. In addition, respiratory epithelial cells exposed to cigarette smoke extract or condensate showed 70% less cilia and shorter cilia compared to control cells (Tamashiro et al., 2009). Mice exposed to cigarette smoke although showed slight increase in ciliary beat frequency at 6 weeks and 3 months, it was significantly reduced at 6 months and these mice also showed significant loss of tracheal ciliated cells (Simet et al., 2010). Decreased number of cilia, reduced ciliary function combined with hypersecretion of mucin, increased viscoelasticity of secreted mucus in COPD patients can lead to airways obstruction and promote persistence of trapped pathogens in the airways(Rose and Voynow, 2006; Voynow et al., 2006). Persistence of bacteria or viruses can further increase production of mucus in the airways (Baginski et al., 2006).

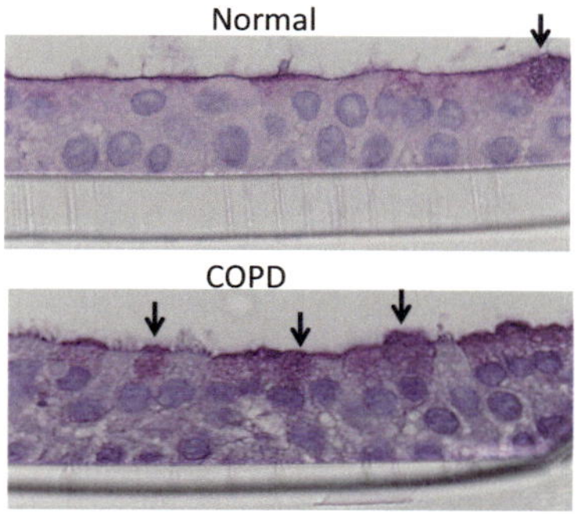

Fig. 1. Airway epithelial cells isolated from COPD patient cultured at air/liquid interface show more goblet cells (arrows) than the similarly grown normal airway epithelial cells.

Another feature that is frequently noted in airways of COPD patients is squamous metaplasia (Araya et al., 2007) and it correlates with the severity of airway obstruction (Cosio et al., 1978). The airway epithelium exposed to cigarette smoke responds by secreting TGF-β (de Boer et al., 1998), which is required for repair of injured epithelium and maintain homeostasis. However, chronic exposure to cigarette smoke can induce sustained production of TGF-β and increased TGF-β activation leading to expression of the β6 integrin, a TGF-β responsive gene (Wang et al., 1996). This in turn contributes to a phenotypic switch from columnar ciliated to squamous epithelium (Masui et al., 1986a; Masui et al., 1986b). Squamous epithelial cells secrete increased amounts of IL-1β, which acts as a paracrine factor with adjacent airway fibroblasts to further activate TGF-β (Araya et al., 2006), thereby increasing squamous metaplasia and further contributing to impaired barrier function and persistence of inhaled pathogens.

In our laboratory, we observed that cultured airway epithelial cells isolated from COPD patients show goblet cell metaplasia, decreased number of ciliated cells (Figure 1), and increased MMP activity suggesting that epigenetic changes that occur *in vivo* are maintained even when cells are expanded *ex vivo* (Schneider et al., 2010). COPD epithelial cells also showed increased viral load following rhinovirus challenge compared to normal cells. Similarly, we also found that elastase/LPS exposed mice which show typical features of COPD, including emphysema, airway remodeling, diffuse lung inflammation and goblet cell hypertrophy, also showed increased persistence of virus compared to normal mice following rhinovirus challenge and majority of the virus particles were observed in the airway epithelium (Sajjan et al., 2009). Rinovirus infection increased mucin expression further in these mice. Since goblet cells are the target for rhinovirus infection (Lachowicz-Scroggins et al., 2010) we suggest that COPD airway epithelial cultures which have increased number of goblet cells are more susceptible to rhinovirus infection than the controls. Patients with COPD, cystic fibrosis and asthma show goblet cell metaplasia and this may be one of the reasons these patients are more susceptible to rhinovirus infection. In addition, airway epithelial mucins also interact with several other respiratory pathogens including *Pseudomonas aeruginosa, Staphylococcus aureus, Heamophilus influenza, Streptococcus pneumonia, Burkholderia cenocepacia*, influenza virus, adenovirus and coronavirus (Landry et al., 2006; Matrosovich and Klenk, 2003; Plotkowski et al., 1993; Ryan et al., 2001; Sajjan and Forstner, 1992; Sajjan et al., 1992; Walters et al., 2002). The bound pathogens which are cleared under normal conditions, persist in the airway lumen when the mucociliary clearance is impaired and initiate inflammatory response and damage the airway epithelium.

2.2 Junctional adherens complexes and airway epithelial permeability

Epithelial permeability is maintained through the cooperation of two mutually exclusive structural components: Tight junctions and adherence junctions on the lateral membranes (Pohl et al., 2009). While tight junctions regulate the transport of solutes and ions across epithelia, adherence junctions mediate cell to cell adhesion (Hartsock and Nelson, 2008; Schneeberger and Lynch, 2004; Shin et al., 2006). Under homeostatic conditions, these intercellular junctions prevent inhaled pathogens and also serve as signaling platforms that regulate gene expression, cell proliferation and differentiation (Balda and Matter, 2009; Koch and Nusrat, 2009). Therefore disassociation or sustained insult that affects junctional complex will disrupt not only barrier function, but also prevent normal repair of airway epithelium. Compared to control nonsmokers, airway epithelium is leaky, hyperproliferative and abnormally differentiated in smokers (Hogg and Timens, 2009). Consistent with this observation, various *in vivo* and *in vitro* studies showed that cigarette smoke increases airway epithelial permeability (Boucher et al., 1980; Gangl et al., 2009; Olivera et al., 2007; Serikov et al., 2006). Recently, transcriptome analysis of airway epithelial cells from normal and COPD patients revealed global down-regulation of physiological tight junction complex gene expression (Shaykhiev et al., 2011). Further, normal airway epithelial cells exposed to cigarette smoke extract also showed similar down-regulation of genes related to tight junction complex. This was associated with decreased expression of PTEN and FOXO3A, a transcriptional factor in the PTEN pathway, suggesting that cigarette smoke down-regulates expression of apical junctional complex genes by modulating PTEN signaling pathway. Consistent with this notion, cigarette smoke in combination with IL-1β has been shown to induce disassembly of tight junction complex in endothelial cells by suppressing PTEN activity (Barbieri et al., 2008). Chen et al showed that cigarette smoke also alters epithelial permeability by disrupting cell polarity via activation of EGFR, dissociation of β-catenin and E-cadherin from adherence junctional complex and redistribution of apical MUC1 membrane bound mucin to cytoplasm (Chen et al., 2010). In a homestatic epithelium, β-catenin cooperates with E-cadherin to form apical junctional complex and maintain cell polarity (Xu and Kimelman, 2007). In airway regeneration or oncogenic formation β-catenin translocates to nucleus, and activates canonical Wnt signaling pathway (Mazieres et al., 2005; Tian et al., 2009). Similar to β-catenin, the cytoplasmic tail of MUC1 also supports structural barrier during homeostasis (Chen et al., 2010). Since cigarette smoke causes aberrant activation of both EGFR and canonical Wnt/β-catenin signaling (Khan et al., 2008; Lemjabbar et al., 2003), it is plausible that chronic cigarette smoke exposure decreases barrier function and promote microbial invasion of airway epithelium.

2.3 Antimicrobial products of airway epithelium

In addition to acting as a physical barrier, airway epithelial cells also secrete antimicrobial substances, which include enzymes, protease inhibitors, oxidants and antimicrobial peptides. Lysozyme is an enzyme found in airway epithelial secretions and exerts antimicrobial effect against wide range of gram-positive bacteria by degrading peptidoglycan layer (Ibrahim et al., 2002). Lysozyme is also effective against gram-negative bacteria in the presence of lactoferrin, which disrupts the outer membrane allowing lysozyme to gain access to peptidoglycan layer (Ellison and Giehl, 1991). Lactoferrin is an iron-chelator and inhibit microbial growth by sequestering iron which is essential for microbial respiration (Ganz, 2002). Lactoferrin also display antiviral activity against both RNA and DNA viruses either by inhibiting binding of virus to host cells or by binding to virus itself (van der Strate et al., 2001; Laube et al., 2006). Lactoferrin levels increase in response to bacterial and viral infections. Epithelial cells produce protease inhibitors, such as secretory leukoprotease inhibitor (SLPI), elastase inhibitor, α1-antiprotease and antichymotrypsin. These protease inhibitors mitigate the effects of proteases expressed by pathogens and recruited innate immune cells. Administration of SLPI decreased the levels of IL-8 and elastase activity in airway secretion of cystic fibrosis patients (McElvaney et al., 1992).

Human beta defensins (hBD) are the most abundant antimicrobial peptides expressed on the surface of airway epithelium and are effective against wide range of bacteria and viruses (Ganz, 2003; Kota et al., 2008; McCray and Bentley, 1997). While hBD1 is constitutively expressed, hBD2 to hBD4 expression is induced by LPS via NF-κB activation and also by IL-1 (Becker et al., 2000; Singh et al., 1998). hBD2 is induced by *P. aeruginosa* infection in normal but not in cystic fibrosis airway epithelia (Dauletbaev et al., 2002). Environmental factors such as air pollutants decrease defensin gene expression in the airways (Laube et al., 2006). In CF airway epithelia activity of hBD2 is also decreased due to increased salt concentration (Goldman et al., 1997). Cathelicidins are another class of antimicrobial peptides and LL37 is the only human cathelicidin identified to date. LL37 bind to LPS and inactivate its biological function. Overexpression of human LL37 in CF mouse model increased killing of *P. aeruginosa* and reduced the ability of this bacterium to colonize the airways (Bals et al., 1998).

Airway epithelial cells also generate oxidants such as nitric oxide (NO) and hydrogen peroxide. Three NO synthases contribute to production of NO in airway epithelia: the constitutively expressed NOS1 and NOS3 and inducible NOS2. Viral infections and pro-inflammatory cytokines induce expression of NOS2 and defective NOS2 expression is responsible for increased viral replication in cystic fibrosis and overexpression of NOS2 provides protection against viral infection (Zheng et al., 2003; Zheng et al., 2004). Hydrogen peroxide is produced by dual oxidase 1 and 2. These belong to a family of NADPH oxidases and are located in the plasma membrane and secrete hydrogen peroxide to extracellular milieu. The dual oxidase-generated hydrogen peroxide in combination with thiocyanate and lactoperoxidase generates the microbicidal oxidant hypothiocyanite , which effectively kills both gram positive and gram negative bacteria and this innate defense mechanism is defective in cystic fibrosis airway epithelium due to impaired transport of thiocyanate (Moskwa et al., 2007).

In COPD patients, levels of lysozyme and SLPI decrease with bacterial infection, while lactoferrin levels remain unchanged (Parameswaran et al., 2011). Lower levels of salivary lysozyme in clinically stable COPD patients correlated with increased risk of exacerbations (Taylor et al., 1995). Reduced lysozyme levels in COPD is thought to be due to degradation by proteases elaborated by bacterial pathogens or neutrophils(Jacquot et al., 1985; Taggart et al., 2001). These proteases also inactivate SLPI (Parameswaran et al., 2009). In addtion, SLPI forms complexes with neutrophil elastase and binds to negatively charged membranes, thus decreasing the levels of SLPI further in the airway secretions during infection. In clinically stable patients however, the levels of SLPI were increased compared to smokers without COPD and never smokers (Tsoumakidou et al., 2010). In contrast, hBD2 was absent in COPD patients. Herr et al showed that hBD2 is significantly reduced in pharyngeal wash and suptum of current or former smokers compared to non-smokers, and exposure of airway epithelium to cigarette smoke *in vitro* inhibited induction of HBD2 by bacteria (Herr et al., 2009). Recently, we showed that COPD airway epithelial cells show a trend in decreased expression of NOS2 and Duox oxidases and this was associated with impaired clearance of rhinovirus (Schneider et al., 2010).

3. Innate immune receptors of airway epithelium

Airway epithelium in addition to providing a physical barrier, it also plays a pivotal role in recognition of pathogens and releasing appropriate chemokine and cytokines to initiate an inflammatory response. This inflammatory response includes recruitment of phagocytes to clear pathogens that are not cleared by barrier function of epithelium, and immune cells, such as dendritic cells and lymphocytes that initiate adaptive immune response. Airway epithelium recognizes pathogens or pathogen associated molecular patterns (PAMPS) by innate immune receptors also known as pattern recognition receptors (PRRs), which are germ-line encoded receptors. One of best characterized PRRs are Toll-like receptors (TLRs)(Akira et al., 2001; Medzhitov, 2001).

3.1 Toll-like receptors

TLRs are type I transmembrane receptors with an extracellular domain that contains leucine-rich-repeat motifs, a transmembrane domain and a cytoplasmic domain known as the toll/interleukin-1 receptor (TIR) homology domain (Hoffmann, 2003) (Figure 2). To date thirteen TLRs have been identified in mammalian system. Only TLRs1 to 10 are expressed in humans. TLRs1, -2, -4, -5 and -6 are expressed on the cell surface and TLRs3, -7,- 8 and -9 are expressed in the endosomes, lysozomes and the endoplastic reticulum. (Kawai and Akira, 2009). TLRs recognize a wide range of PAMPS- lipoproteins by TLRs 1, -2, and -6 (Aliprantis et al., 1999; Schwandner et al., 1999; Takeuchi et al., 2001; Takeuchi et al., 2002), LPS by TLR4 (Poltorak et al., 1998), flagella by TLR5 (Hayashi et al., 2001), DNA by TLR9 (Hemmi et al., 2000), and RNA by TLR3, -7 and -8 (Alexopoulou et al., 2001; Diebold et al., 2004; Heil et al., 2004). TLR4 also recognizes respiratory syncytial virus (Kurt-Jones et al., 2000).

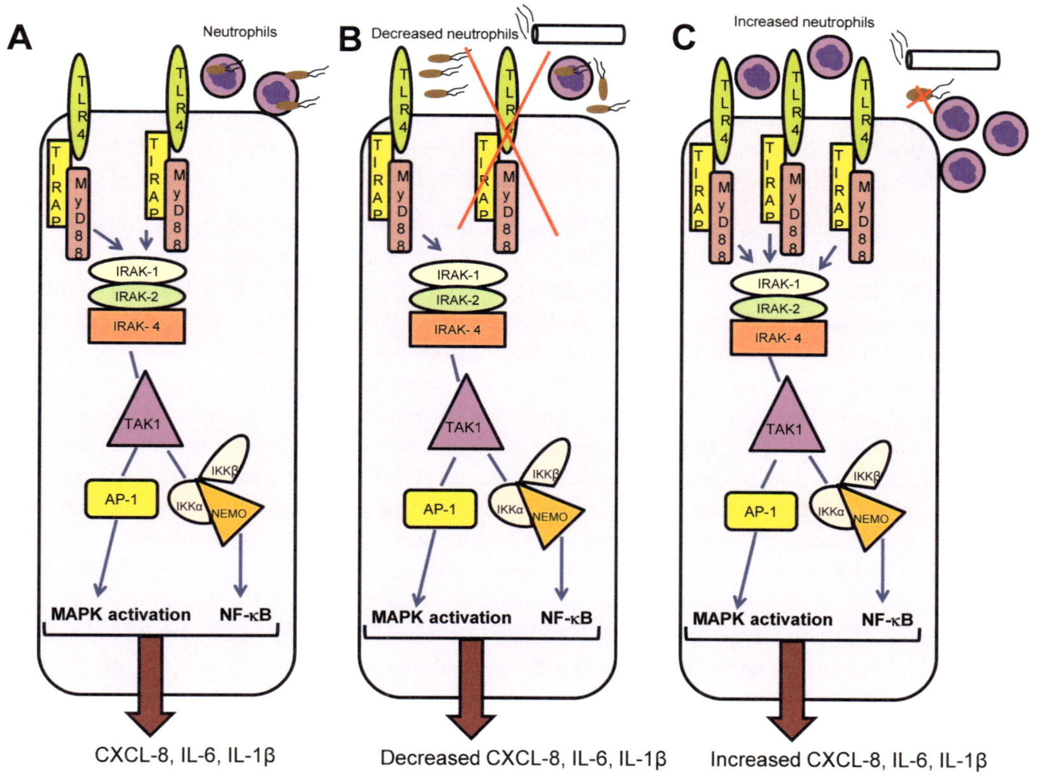

Fig. 2. Impact of cigarette smoke on persistence of bacteria and inflammation. Under homeostasis, TLR4 recognizes infecting bacteria and activates both MAP kinase and NF-kB pathway to stimulate normal levels of CXCL-8, IL-6 and IL-1β to recruit neutrophils, which clear bacteria. Decreased expression of TLR4 caused by acute exposure to cigarette smoke attenuates release of CXCL-8, IL-6 and IL-1β, there by decreasing the neutrophil infiltration and increasing the bacterial persistence. Under chronic exposure as noted in COPD patients, if the TLR4 expression is increased, then chemokine and cytokine expression is increased leading to decreased bacteria coupled with increased inflammation.

TLRs initiate signaling by MyD (myeloid differentiation primary-response protein) 88-dependent and -independent pathways. Except for TLR3, all TLRs initiate signaling by MyD-88-depnedent pathway to activate NF-κB. MyD88 is located in the cytoplasm and is similar to

TLR in structure and has an N-terminal death domain, an intermediary domain and C-terminal TIR domain. Upon recognition of PAMPs by TLRs, the TIR domain of TLR interacts with TIR domain of MyD88 directly or indirectly via MyD88-adaptor like protein (MAL)/TIR adaptor protein (TIRAP)(Horng et al., 2002; Li et al., 2005). TLR5, -7, -8 and -9 does not require TIRAP to initiate signaling events that leads to NF-κB activation (Horng et al., 2002). Association of MyD88 to TLR leads to recruitment of IL-1R associated kinase (IRAK)-4, IRAK-1, TNFR-associated factor 6 (TRAF6), which then through a number of kinases activates NF-κB and AP-1 and stimulates expression of CXCL-8, IL-6, IL-1β and TNF-α (Adachi et al., 1998; Mukaida et al., 1990; Jeong and Lee, 2011). TLR4 also signals via MyD88-independent pathway and the first supporting evidence came from the studies on MyD88 knockout mice, which failed to respond normally to TLR2, -5, -7 and -9 ligands, but not to TLR4 (Kawai et al., 1999). Later TLR4 endocytosed upon binding to LPS was shown to signal through TIR-domain-containing adapter-inducing interferon (IFN)-β (TRIF) pathway similar to TLR3 (Alexopoulou et al., 2001; Hoebe et al., 2003; Kagan et al., 2008). TLR2 was shown to be internalized and stimulate type I interferon (IFN) response by MyD88-dependent pathway in virus-, but not bacteria infected inflammatory monocytes (Barbalat et al., 2009).

The airway epithelium expresses all 10 TLRs, but the expression of TLR2 to TLR6 is stronger than the others. Expression of TLRs7 through -10 is variable depending on type of cells used (Mayer et al., 2007; Platz et al., 2004; Sha et al., 2004). Expression of TLRs 1 through -6 and -9 on the cell surface was confirmed by flow cytometry (Greene et al., 2005). However the signaling from these TLRs depends on the expression of adaptor molecules and co-receptors. Primary airway epithelial cells are hyporesponsive to LPS despite expressing TLR4 and this is because of reduced surface expression of co-receptor CD14 and low expression levels of co-stimulatory molecule MD2 (Jia et al., 2004). This may be necessary to restrict TLR4 activation under unstimulated conditions to prevent chronic inflammation of airways that is constantly exposed to inhaled bacteria and endotoxin. On the contrary, LPS was shown to activate TLR4 signaling in small airway and alveolar epithelial cells even though the TLR4 was localized to cytoplasmic compartment (Guillot et al., 2004). More recently John et al attributed chronic colonization of bacteria in CF airways to decreased expression of TLR4 in CF airway epithelial cells (John et al., 2010). TLR2, which is expressed on the apical surface of polarized airway cells is mobilized into an apical lipid raft receptor complex following *P. aeruginosa* infection and initiate signalling (Soong et al., 2004). TLR5 recgonizes flagella of *P. aeruginosa* and *Burkholderia cenocepacia* and activate NF-κB (Adamo et al., 2004; Urban et al., 2004; Zhang et al., 2005). *Haemophilus influenzae* traverses polarized airway epithelial cells by interacting with TLR2, which then activates p38 mitogen activated protein (MAP) kinase and TGF-β Signalling(Beisswenger et al., 2007). TLR3 recognizes double stranded (ds)-RNA, an intermediate generated during RNA virus replication and elicits chemokine and type I IFN responses by MyD88- independent signaling mechanism (Gern et al., 2003; Wang et al., 2009). Upon ligation of ds-RNA, TRIF and TRAM (TRIF-related adaptor molecule) are recruited to TIR domain of TLR3 and TRAM acts as a bridge between TLR and TRIF and this allows activation of TRIF-dependent signaling leading to activation of IRF3 via IKKε/TBK-1 to stimulate IFN production or activation of NF-κB via IKKα/IKKβ to stimulate CXCL-8 expression (Kawai and Akira, 2008). The recognition of double-stranded RNA by TLR3 also increases expression of hBD2 (Duits et al., 2003). Viral or bacterial infection transcriptionally upregulates TLR3 expression (Liu et al., 2007; Sajjan et al., 2006; Wang et al., 2009; Xing et al., 2011), thereby increasing viral induced cytokine and chemokine responses further. Stimulation of TLR2 or TLR3 also induces mucin expression by activating MAP kinases and inducing EGF receptor signaling (Chen et al., 2004; Kohri et al., 2002; Li et al., 1997; Zhu et al., 2009). MUC1, a transmembrane mucin is a negative regulator of TLRs and therefore may play an important role in limiting TLR- induced inflammatory responses (Ueno et al., 2008).

There are conflicting reports with regards to expression of TLRs and their role in innate immune responses in patients with COPD. Airway epithelial cells from patients with severe COPD showed decreased expression of TLR4, but not TLR2 (MacRedmond et al., 2007). In contrast, recently Pace et al observed increased neutrophils and decreased apoptosis of neutrophils in the bronchoalveolar lavage and increased expression of TLR4 in airway epithelium of COPD patients providing evidence that increased TLR4 may contribute to airway neutrophilia in COPD (Pace et al., 2011). Pace et al also demonstrated increased TLR4 expression and concurrent increased CXCL-8 in response to LPS challenge in cigarette smoke exposed airway epithelial cells(Pace et al., 2008), while other investigators showed decreased TLR4 expression which was associated with reduced CXCL-8 and hBD2 production (Kulkarni et al., 2010; MacRedmond et al., 2007). Our preliminary studies involving primary airway epithelial cells from COPD patients suggested heightened expression of CXCL-8 in responses to *P. aeruginosa* infection compared to normal airway epithelial cells (Ganesan and Sajjan, unpublished results). However, role of TLR in this context is yet to be established. Whether TLR4 expression is decreased or increased it has important implications in COPD airway inflammation and obstruction (Figure 2). The decreased expression of TLR4 may lead to decreased innate immune responses and increased persistence of infecting organism. On the other hand increased expression of TLR4 increases neutrophil recruitment and mucus production in response to bacterial or viral infection, thereby leading to increased airways inflammation and obstruction.

3.2 RIG-I like receptors

Another family of PRRs that play a role in innate defense mechanisms of airway epithelial cells is retinoic acid inducible (RIG)-I like receptors (RLR). This family of PRRs includes RIG-I, MDA-5 (melanoma differentiation associated protein 5) and LGP-2 (Laboratory of genetics and physiology 2). RLRs are the primary sensor molecules for detection of viral RNA in the cytoplasm (Meylan and Tschopp, 2006; Sun et al., 2006). Both RIG-I and MDA-5 contain a caspase recruitment domain (CARD) and a RNA helicase domain (Kang et al., 2002; Yoneyama et al., 2005; Yoneyama et al., 2004). On the other hand, LPG-2 has only RNA helicase domain but not CARD domain, which is required for recruiting adaptor protein MAVS (also known as VISA, Cardiff)(Yoneyama et al., 2005). Therefore recognition of viral RNA by RIG-I and MDA-5 leads to IFN or chemokine response, and LPG-2 suppresses this response (Yoneyama et al., 2005). RIG-I and MDA-5 recognize different RNA species. RIG-I recognizes single stranded (ss)RNA viruses, such as influenza virus, paramyxoviruses and deficiency in RIG-I increases the susceptibility of mice to RNA viruses (Kato et al., 2005). RIG-I specifically binds to the 5′-triphosphate moiety, the signature of which is exposed in the process of viral entry or replication. The host RNA which loses 5′triphosphate moiety during processing is therefore not recognized by RIG-I preventing cytokine and chemokine response due to self-recognition. RIG-I also recognizes short dsRNA (<1 kb) in 5′triphosphate-independent manner and induces IFN responses (Kato et al., 2008). On the other hand, MDA-5 recognizes long dsRNA that is >1 kb. Since viruses from picornaviridea family including rhinovirus generate long dsRNA in infected cells, innate immune responses to these viruses depends on recognition of viral RNA by MDA-5 (Kato et al., 2006; Wang et al., 2009). Mice deficient in MDA-5 show increased inflammatory response, delayed IFN response and significantly increased viral load up to 48 h after rhinovirus infection (Wang et al., 2011) . Both RIG-I and MDA-5 uses a common adaptor protein called interferon beta promoter stimulator-1 (IPS-1, also known as MAVS, VISA, CARDIF)(Kawai et al., 2005; Meylan et al., 2005; Seth et al., 2005; Xu et al., 2005). IPS-1 has a CARD domain which is homologous to RIG-I and MDA-5 and has a transmembrane domain at its C-terminal end that spans the mitochondrial membrane (Seth et al., 2005). IPS-1 after binding to RIG-I or MDA-5 through CARD-CARD interaction, activates IRF3 and NF-κB via TBK1/IKKε and RIP-1/IKKα/IKKβ respectively. IPS-1 also interacts with receptor-interacting protein-1 (RIP-1), which is a death domain and is implicated in virus infection-induced IFN expression (Balachandran et al., 2004). However IPS-1 interaction with RIP-1 via the non-CARD region facilitates NF-κB activation, rather than IRF3 activation. Therefore IPS-1 regulates both IRF3 and NF-κB activation upon binding to RIG-I or MDA-5. IPS-1-deficient mice fail to activate IRF3 and NF-κB, with concomitant loss of type I IFN and inflammatory cytokine induction after viral infection and show increased persistence of virus (Kawai and Akira, 2008). Recently, cigarette smoke extract was demonstrated to inhibit RIG-I-stimulated innate immune responses to influenza infection in bronchial organ culture model (Wu et al., 2011). Exposure to cigarette smoke extract also interfered with STAT1 activation by IFN-γ, a type II interferon which stimulates expression of various antiviral proteins (Modestou et al., 2010). Further, cigarette smoke also attenuated the inhibitor effect of IFN-γ on RSV mRNA and protein expression. Eddleston et al demonstrated that exposure of airway epithelial cells to cigarette smoke extract suppressed mRNA induction of CXCL-10 and IFN-β by human rhinovirus and also viral dsRNA mimic polyinosinic:polycytidylic acid (poly I:C) (Eddleston et al., 2011). This was found to be due to decrease in activation of the IFN-STAT-1 and SAP-JNK pathways. Inhibition of antiviral responses, in particular IFN and CXCL-10 responses appear to be due to acute exposure to cigarette smoke that occurs *in vitro*, because the airway epithelial cells obtained from COPD patients showed antiviral responses to rhinovirus infection which was in fact significantly higher than the cells obtained from non-smokers (Schneider et al., 2010). Similar to our observations, mice exposed to cigarette smoke and poly I:C or influenza virus showed increased IFN responses and this was attributed to pathogenesis of COPD (Kang et al., 2008).

3.3 NOD-like receptors

Nod-like receptors (NLR) are a family of proteins and sense microbial signatures in the cytosol. There are at least 22 identified NLRs in humans, although only few of them have been functionally characterized. All of them have a central nucleotide binding domain and C-terminal leucin-rich repeat domain, which possibly mediate ligand binding. In addition, they also contain different N-terminal effector domains such as CARD domain, pyrin domains or baculovirus inhibitor repeats and thus activate diverse downstream signaling pathways (Chen et al., 2009; Fritz et al., 2006). The most widely studied among the CARD containing NLRs are NOD1 and NOD2. NOD1 primarily recognizes peptidoglycan (PGN) derivative, γ-D-glutamyl-mesodiaminopimelic acid from gram-negative bacteria (Chamaillard et al., 2003; Girardin et al., 2003a), whereas, NOD2 is considered as a general sensor of PGN through muramyl dipeptide (Girardin et al., 2003b). Upon recognizing PGN, both NOD1 and NOD2 activate NF-κB-mediated proinflammatory response via RIP-2 (Hasegawa et al., 2008). Both NOD1 and NOD2 are highly expressed in immune and inflammatory cells (Fritz et al., 2005; Kanneganti et al., 2007). These two NODs are also expressed in airway epithelium and are induced by bacterial stimuli (Bogefors et al., 2010; Mayer et al., 2007; Opitz et al., 2004; Travassos et al., 2005). NOD1 and NOD2 contribute to innate immune responses to different bacteria including *Pseudomonas aeruginosa, Chlamydia pneumonia, Haemophilus influenza* and *L. pneumophila* both *in vivo* and *in vitro* (Clarke et al., 2010; Frutuoso et al., 2010; Shimada et al., 2009; Zola et al., 2008).

NOD2 not only recognizes bacterial peptidoglycan, but also viral ssRNA. NOD2 deficiency results in impaired type I IFN expression *in vitro* upon stimulation with viral ssRNA (Sabbah et al., 2009). This was dependent on NOD2 interaction with IPS-1 and activation of IRF3, but not on activation of RIP-2. NOD2 deficient mice were also found to be more susceptible to infection with respiratory syncytial virus and influenza virus than the wild-type mice.

Pyrin domain containing NLRs are normally called as NLRP. There are 14 members in this NLR subfamily. At least NLRP1-3 form multiprotein complex named "inflammasomes" which consists one or two NLRs, an adaptor molecule ASC (apoptosis-associated speck-like protein containing a CARD), and caspase-1(Martinon et al., 2002). Inflammasomes respond to several PAMPS or DAMPS and regulate caspase-1 mediated cell death called pyroptosis and production of IL-1β and IL-18 at post-transcriptional level. Therefore, unlike other cytokines, IL-1β production requires two signals. Signal I is often provided by TLRs which activates NF-κB dependent pro-IL-1β, and signal II comes from inflammasomes, which mediate caspase 1-dependent cleavage of pro-IL-1β to its mature form. The activators of NLRP3 are microbial RNA, bacterial pore forming toxins, certain types of DNA and MDP (Kanneganti et al., 2006; Mariathasan et al., 2006; Martinon et al., 2004; Meixenberger et al., 2010; Muruve et al., 2008). Accordingly, NLRP3 null mice were shown to be susceptible to influenza virus, *Streptococcus pneumoniae* and *K. pneumonia* infection (Kanneganti, 2010; Allen et al., 2009; Ichinohe et al., 2010; Thomas et al., 2009). In addition NLRP3 is also activated by necrotic cells, uric acid metabolites, ATP, biglycan, hyaluronan that might be released after tissue injury (Babelova et al., 2009; Iyer et al., 2009; Mariathasan et al., 2006; Martinon et al., 2006; Yamasaki et al., 2009).

In addition to NLRP, NLRC4 (NLR family CARD domain containing) and NAIP5 (NLR family, BIRdomain conaining) also form inflammasomes. While NAIP is expressed in both lung macrophages and epithelial cells, NLRC4 is expressed only in macrophages (Diez et al., 2000; Vinzing et al., 2008). NLRC4 inflammasome recognizes *L. pneumophila* and *P. aeruginosa* flagellin present in the host cytosol, independently of TLR5 (Franchi et al., 2006; Miao et al., 2006). NAIP controls intracellular replication of *L. pneumophila* depending on the recognition of flagellin (Vinzing et al., 2008).

The widely expressed NLRX1 (NLR family member X1) is the only NLR receptor that is localized to mitochondria and it negatively regulates RIG-I and MDA-5 receptors. NLRX-1 mediates production of reactive oxygen species upon bacterial infection (Moore et al., 2008; Tattoli et al., 2008) and decreased dsRNA-stimulated IFN response.

Although, there is no evidence that NLRs play a role in innate immune responses to bacterial or viral infection in COPD so far, the emerging literature indicate inflammasome forming NLRs may contribute to COPD pathogenesis. Inhaled cigarette smoke, oxidative stress, necrotic cell death, hypoxia, hypercapnia may cause tissue injury and release of DAMPs (uric acid, ATP) and this in turn activates NLRP3 inflammasome (Wanderer, 2008). Consistent with this notion, uric acid concentration was increased in the bronchoalveolar lavage of COPD patients (Wanderer, 2008). COPD patients also had significantly increased amounts of IL-1β and this correlated with severity of the disease(Sapey et al., 2009). Mice exposed to cigarette smoke also showed increased IL-1β in their lungs (Doz et al., 2008) and finally mice overexpressing mature IL-1β in epithelial cells showed typical feature of COPD including emphysema, lung inflammation with increased neutrophils and macrophages and airway fibrosis (Lappalainen et al., 2005). ASC (inflammasome adaptor protein) null mice showed attenuated inflammation after exposing to elastase and less uric acid. Elastase-induced inflammation was significantly reduced in wild-type mice treated with uricase or treated with IL-1R antagonist (Couillin et al., 2009). All these evidences suggest contribution of inflammasome forming NLRP3 to COPD pathogenesis.

4. Innate immunity and co-infections

Nontypeable *H. influenzae* (NTHi), *S. Pneumoniae* and *P. aeruginosa* are detectable in lower airways of appproximatley 25 to 50% of clinically stable COPD patients (Sethi and Murphy, 2008). Chronic colonization can alter the responses of airway epithelial cells and other innate and adaptive immune cells to subsequent viral or bacterial infections leading to increased severity of disease. Exacerbations due to concurrent or sequential infections was shown to be associated with increased severity of disease at least in one-quarter of COPD patient population (Papi et al., 2006; Sethi et al., 2006; Wilkinson et al., 2006). Risk of secondary bacterial infection following a viral infection dates back to 19th century, when cases of pneumonia correlated with influenza (flu) epidemic (McCullers, 2006). Influenza infection increases risk of secondary bacterial infection by increasing binding or invasion of bacterial pathogen to airway epithelial cells, desensitizing innate immune receptors such as TLRs, and causing immunosuppression by increasing glucocorticosteriod expression (Beadling and Slifka, 2004; Hament et al., 1999; Jamieson et al., 2010; McCullers, 2006; Seki et al., 2004; Sun and Metzger, 2008). Respiratory syncytial virus infection increased persistence of *P. aeruginosa* in mice and increased *P. aeruginosa* and NTHi binding to airway epithelial cells (de Vrankrijker et al., 2009; Jiang et al., 1999; Van Ewijk et al., 2007). Respiratory syncytial virus also increased persistence of NTHi by dysregulating the expression of β-defensin in chinchilla model of respiratory infection (McGillivary et al., 2009). Rhinovirus which causes common cold, in combination with *S. pnuemoniae* was associated with severe cases of community-acquired pneumonia in children (Honkinen et al., 2011). Various *in vitro* studies showed that rhinoviruses also increase bacterial binding to airway epithelial cells by increasing the expression of bacterial receptors on airway epithelial cells or by facilitating invasion of cells by bacteria (Ishizuka et al., 2003; Passariello et al., 2006). We demonstrated that rhinovirus infection also increases paracellular permeability and promote bacterial traversal across mucociliary- differentiated airway epithelium (Sajjan et al., 2008). Rhinovirus infection also decreases bacterial PAMPS-induced proinflammatory response by desensitizing TLRs (Oliver et al., 2008).

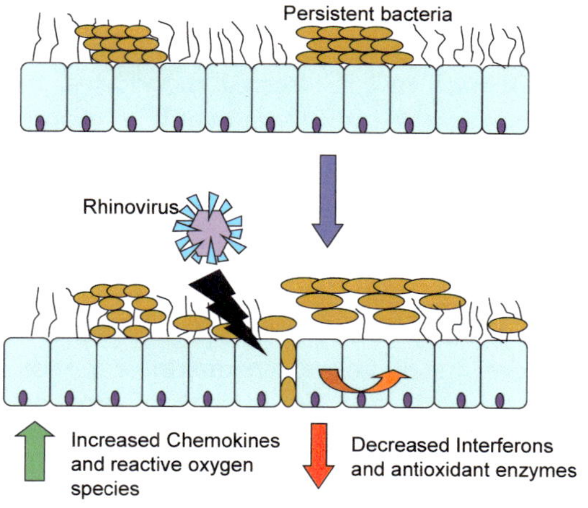

Fig. 3. COPD airway epithelial cells are impaired in clearing infecting bacteria. This leads to colonization of bacteria on the apical surface of airway epithelium. Subsequent rhinovirus infection disrupts barrier function and promotes traversal and interaction of bacteria with basolateral receptors leading to exaggerated chemokine response. At the same time COPD airway epithelial cells also show increased generation of reactive oxygen species and attenuated expression of antioxidant enzymes resulting in increased oxidative stress. This in turn suppresses interferon (antiviral) response stimulated by secondary rhinovirus infection. Together this may lead to persistence of bacteria and virus, and increased inflammation.

Impact of secondary viral or bacterial infection in patients colonized with bacteria is being increasingly recognized in recent years. For instance, despite chronic colonization with *P. aeruginosa*, cystic fibrosis patients show exacerbations periodically and some incidences are associated with acquiring secondary viral or bacterial infections (Ong et al., 1989; Ramsey et al., 1989; Wat et al., 2008). Similarly, in COPD patients who are chronically colonized with NTHi, exacerbations were associated with acquisition of new strain of NTHi, other species of bacteria or respiratory virus (Murphy, 2000; Murphy et al., 2008; Murphy et al., 2007; Papi et al., 2006; Sykes et al., 2007; Wilson, 2000). Recently, we showed that secondary bacterial infection in primary cystic fibrosis airway epithelial cells preinfected with *P. aeruginosa* increases C-X-C chemokine responses by increasing the load of planktonic bacteria which are more pro-inflammatory than their counterpart biofilm bacteria and also increased paracellular invasion of bacteria in differentiated airway epithelial cells (Chattoraj et al., 2011b). We also demonstrated that cystic fibrosis, but not normal airway epithelial cells infected with bacteria show suppressed type I IFN response to subsequent rhinovirus infection (Chattoraj et al., 2011a). This was due to increased oxidative stress in cystic fibrosis airway epithelial cells. Airway epithelial cells from COPD patients show increased oxidative stress similar to cystic fibrosis patients. Therefore we expect that bacterial preinfection may suppress innate immune responses to subsequent virus infection in COPD cells. Consistent with this notion, our preliminary studies indicate that infection with *P. aeruginosa* or NTHi infection increases oxidative stress further and decreases expression of antioxidant genes in COPD airway epithelial cells. In addition, we also observed suppression of IFN response in COPD airway epithelial cells infected with bacteria to subsequent rhinovirus infection (unpublished observations). Similar to our observations, LPS treatment was demonstrated to suppress IFN-β production in response to dsRNA in mice as well as in monocytes and macrophages (Piao et al., 2009; Sly et al., 2009). This was due to increased expression of SHIP, a MPA kinase phosphatase in LPS treated monocytes. In airway epithelial cells however, *P. aeruginosa* infection induced suppression of IFN response to rhinovirus infection was not due to increased expression of SHIP, but rather due to decreased Akt phosphorylation (Chattoraj et al 2011) which is required for maximal activation of IRF3 (Dong et al., 2008; Sarkar et al., 2004). Previously, we have shown that expression of IFN response to rhinovirus infection requires activation of IRF3 in airway epithelial cells (Wang et al., 2009). Based on these experimental evidences, it is possible that 30% of COPD patients who are chronically colonized with *NTHi* or *P. aeruginosa* in their lower airways may show suppressed antiviral responses and increased chemokine expression (Figure 3). This may lead to increased lung inflammation and progression of lung disease in COPD patients following exacerbation due to co-infections.

5. Conclusion

The airway epithelium contributes significantly to innate immune system in the lungs. It acts as a physical barrier that protects against inhaled substances and pathogens. Airway epithelial cells also express plethora of innate immune receptors which recognizes both PAMPS and DAMPS and stimulate appropriate responses to either clear the infecting organism and to repair of injured epithelium. However in COPD, chronic exposure to cigarette smoke or environmental hazards causes airway remodeling and also modulate innate immune responses of airway epithelial cells to infection (Figure 4). This results in impaired clearance of infecting organisms and aberrant cytokine and growth factor expression and increased lung inflammation leading to progression of lung disease.

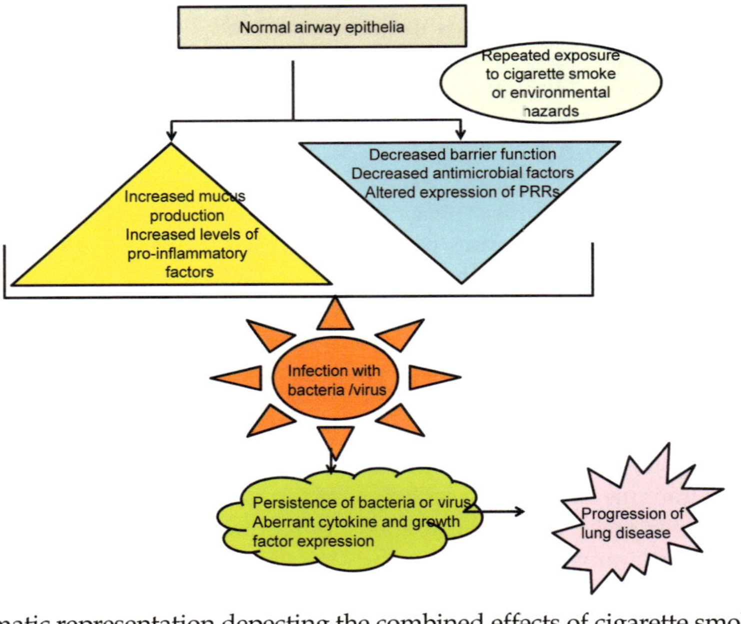

Fig. 4. A schematic representation depecting the combined effects of cigarette smoke or other environmental hazards and bacterial infection on the progression of lung disease in COPD

6. Acknowledgements

This work was supported by NIH AT4793 and HL897720 to U.S. We thank Marisa Lynn for assisting with processing cell cultures for histology and Adam Comstock for his assistance in culturing primary epithelial cells.

7. References

Adachi, O., Kawai, T., Takeda, K., Matsumoto, M., Tsutsui, H., Sakagami, M., Nakanishi, K., and Akira, S. (1998). Targeted disruption of the MyD88 gene results in loss of IL-1- and IL-18-mediated function. Immunity *9*, 143-150.

Adamo, R., Sokol, S., Soong, G., Gomez, M.I., and Prince, A. (2004). Pseudomonas aeruginosa flagella activate airway epithelial cells through asialoGM1 and toll-like receptor 2 as well as toll-like receptor 5. Am J Respir Cell Mol Biol *30*, 627-634.

Adcock, I.M., Caramori, G., and Barnes, P.J. (2011). Chronic obstructive pulmonary disease and lung cancer: new molecular insights. Respiration *81*, 265-284.

Akira, S., Takeda, K., and Kaisho, T. (2001). Toll-like receptors: critical proteins linking innate and acquired immunity. Nat Immunol *2*, 675-680.

Alexopoulou, L., Holt, A.C., Medzhitov, R., and Flavell, R.A. (2001). Recognition of double-stranded RNA and activation of NF-kappaB by Toll-like receptor 3. Nature *413*, 732-738.

Aliprantis, A.O., Yang, R.B., Mark, M.R., Suggett, S., Devaux, B., Radolf, J.D., Klimpel, G.R., Godowski, P., and Zychlinsky, A. (1999). Cell activation and apoptosis by bacterial lipoproteins through toll-like receptor-2. Science *285*, 736-739.

Allen, I.C., Scull, M.A., Moore, C.B., Holl, E.K., McElvania-TeKippe, E., Taxman, D.J., Guthrie, E.H., Pickles, R.J., and Ting, J.P. (2009). The NLRP3 inflammasome mediates in vivo innate immunity to influenza A virus through recognition of viral RNA. Immunity *30*, 556-565.

Araya, J., Cambier, S., Markovics, J.A., Wolters, P., Jablons, D., Hill, A., Finkbeiner, W., Jones, K., Broaddus, V.C., Sheppard, D., *et al.* (2007). Squamous metaplasia amplifies pathologic epithelial-mesenchymal interactions in COPD patients. J Clin Invest *117*, 3551-3562.

Araya, J., Cambier, S., Morris, A., Finkbeiner, W., and Nishimura, S.L. (2006). Integrin-mediated transforming growth factor-beta activation regulates homeostasis of the pulmonary epithelial-mesenchymal trophic unit. Am J Pathol *169*, 405-415.

Babelova, A., Moreth, K., Tsalastra-Greul, W., Zeng-Brouwers, J., Eickelberg, O., Young, M.F., Bruckner, P., Pfeilschifter, J., Schaefer, R.M., Grone, H.J., *et al.* (2009). Biglycan, a danger signal that activates the NLRP3 inflammasome via toll-like and P2X receptors. J Biol Chem *284*, 24035-24048.

Baginski, T.K., Dabbagh, K., Satjawatcharaphong, C., and Swinney, D.C. (2006). Cigarette smoke synergistically enhances respiratory mucin induction by proinflammatory stimuli. Am J Respir Cell Mol Biol *35*, 165-174.

Balachandran, S., Thomas, E., and Barber, G.N. (2004). A FADD-dependent innate immune mechanism in mammalian cells. Nature *432*, 401-405.

Balda, M.S., and Matter, K. (2009). Tight junctions and the regulation of gene expression. Biochim Biophys Acta *1788*, 761-767.

Bals, R., and Hiemstra, P.S. (2004). Innate immunity in the lung: how epithelial cells fight against respiratory pathogens. Eur Respir J *23*, 327-333.

Bals, R., Wang, X., Zasloff, M., and Wilson, J.M. (1998). The peptide antibiotic LL-37/hCAP-18 is expressed in epithelia of the human lung where it has broad antimicrobial activity at the airway surface. Proc Natl Acad Sci U S A *95*, 9541-9546.

Barbalat, R., Lau, L., Locksley, R.M., and Barton, G.M. (2009). Toll-like receptor 2 on inflammatory monocytes induces type I interferon in response to viral but not bacterial ligands. Nat Immunol *10*, 1200-1207.

Barbieri, S.S., Ruggiero, L., Tremoli, E., and Weksler, B.B. (2008). Suppressing PTEN activity by tobacco smoke plus interleukin-1beta modulates dissociation of VE-cadherin/beta-catenin complexes in endothelium. Arterioscler Thromb Vasc Biol *28*, 732-738.

Beadling, C., and Slifka, M.K. (2004). How do viral infections predispose patients to bacterial infections? Curr Opin Infect Dis *17*, 185-191.

Becker, M.N., Diamond, G., Verghese, M.W., and Randell, S.H. (2000). CD14-dependent lipopolysaccharide-induced beta-defensin-2 expression in human tracheobronchial epithelium. J Biol Chem *275*, 29731-29736.

Beisswenger, C., Coyne, C.B., Shchepetov, M., and Weiser, J.N. (2007). Role of p38 MAP kinase and transforming growth factor-beta signaling in transepithelial migration of invasive bacterial pathogens. J Biol Chem *282*, 28700-28708.

Bhowmik, A., Chahal, K., Austin, G., and Chakravorty, I. (2009). Improving mucociliary clearance in chronic obstructive pulmonary disease. Respir Med *103*, 496-502.

Bogefors, J., Rydberg, C., Uddman, R., Fransson, M., Mansson, A., Benson, M., Adner, M., and Cardell, L.O. (2010). Nod1, Nod2 and Nalp3 receptors, new potential targets in treatment of allergic rhinitis? Allergy *65*, 1222-1226.

Borchers, M.T., Carty, M.P., and Leikauf, G.D. (1999). Regulation of human airway mucins by acrolein and inflammatory mediators. The American journal of physiology *276*, L549-555.

Boucher, R.C., Johnson, J., Inoue, S., Hulbert, W., and Hogg, J.C. (1980). The effect of cigarette smoke on the permeability of guinea pig airways. Lab Invest *43*, 94-100.

Casalino-Matsuda, S.M., Monzon, M.E., Day, A.J., and Forteza, R.M. (2009). Hyaluronan fragments/CD44 mediate oxidative stress-induced MUC5B up-regulation in airway epithelium. Am J Respir Cell Mol Biol *40*, 277-285.

Chamaillard, M., Hashimoto, M., Horie, Y., Masumoto, J., Qiu, S., Saab, L., Ogura, Y., Kawasaki, A., Fukase, K., Kusumoto, S., *et al.* (2003). An essential role for NOD1 in host recognition of bacterial peptidoglycan containing diaminopimelic acid. Nat Immunol *4*, 702-707.

Chattoraj, S.S., Ganesan, S., Faris, A., Comstock, A., Lee, W.M., and Sajjan, U.S. (2011a). Pseudomonas aeruginosa suppresses interferon response to rhinovirus infection in Cystic fibrosis, but not in normal bronchial epithelial cells. Infect Immun 79, 4131-4145.

Chattoraj, S.S., Ganesan, S., Jones, A.M., Helm, J.M., Comstock, A.T., Bright-Thomas, R., LiPuma, J.J., Hershenson, M.B., and Sajjan, U.S. (2011b). Rhinovirus infection liberates planktonic bacteria from biofilm and increases chemokine responses in cystic fibrosis airway epithelial cells. Thorax *66*, 333-339.

Chen, G., Shaw, M.H., Kim, Y.G., and Nunez, G. (2009). NOD-like receptors: role in innate immunity and inflammatory disease. Annu Rev Pathol *4*, 365-398.

Chen, R., Lim, J.H., Jono, H., Gu, X.X., Kim, Y.S., Basbaum, C.B., Murphy, T.F., and Li, J.D. (2004). Nontypeable Haemophilus influenzae lipoprotein P6 induces MUC5AC mucin transcription via TLR2-TAK1-dependent p38 MAPK-AP1 and IKKbeta-IkappaBalpha-NF-kappaB signaling pathways. Biochem Biophys Res Commun *324*, 1087-1094.

Chen, Y.T., Gallup, M., Nikulina, K., Lazarev, S., Zlock, L., Finkbeiner, W., and McNamara, N. (2010). Cigarette smoke induces epidermal growth factor receptor-dependent redistribution of apical MUC1 and junctional beta-catenin in polarized human airway epithelial cells. Am J Pathol *177*, 1255-1264.

Choi, W.I., Syrkina, O., Kwon, K.Y., Quinn, D.A., and Hales, C.A. (2010). JNK activation is responsible for mucus overproduction in smoke inhalation injury. Respir Res *11*, 172.

Clarke, T.B., Davis, K.M., Lysenko, E.S., Zhou, A.Y., Yu, Y., and Weiser, J.N. (2010). Recognition of peptidoglycan from the microbiota by Nod1 enhances systemic innate immunity. Nat Med *16*, 228-231.

Cohen, N.A., Zhang, S., Sharp, D.B., Tamashiro, E., Chen, B., Sorscher, E.J., and Woodworth, B.A. (2009). Cigarette smoke condensate inhibits transepithelial chloride transport and ciliary beat frequency. Laryngoscope *119*, 2269-2274.

Cosio, M., Ghezzo, H., Hogg, J.C., Corbin, R., Loveland, M., Dosman, J., and Macklem, P.T. (1978). The relations between structural changes in small airways and pulmonary-function tests. N Engl J Med *298*, 1277-1281.

Couillin, I., Vasseur, V., Charron, S., Gasse, P., Tavernier, M., Guillet, J., Lagente, V., Fick, L., Jacobs, M., Coelho, F.R., *et al.* (2009). IL-1R1/MyD88 signaling is critical for elastase-induced lung inflammation and emphysema. J Immunol *183*, 8195-8202.

Curran, D.R., and Cohn, L. (2010). Advances in mucous cell metaplasia: a plug for mucus as a therapeutic focus in chronic airway disease. Am J Respir Cell Mol Biol *42*, 268-275.

Dauletbaev, N., Gropp, R., Frye, M., Loitsch, S., Wagner, T.O., and Bargon, J. (2002). Expression of human beta defensin (HBD-1 and HBD-2) mRNA in nasal epithelia of adult cystic fibrosis patients, healthy individuals, and individuals with acute cold. Respiration *69*, 46-51.

de Boer, W.I., van Schadewijk, A., Sont, J.K., Sharma, H.S., Stolk, J., Hiemstra, P.S., and van Krieken, J.H. (1998). Transforming growth factor beta1 and recruitment of macrophages and mast cells in airways in chronic obstructive pulmonary disease. Am J Respir Crit Care Med *158*, 1951-1957.

de Vrankrijker, A.M., Wolfs, T.F., Ciofu, O., Hoiby, N., van der Ent, C.K., Poulsen, S.S., and Johansen, H.K. (2009). Respiratory syncytial virus infection facilitates acute colonization of Pseudomonas aeruginosa in mice. J Med Virol *81*, 2096-2103.

Diamond, G., Legarda, D., and Ryan, L.K. (2000). The innate immune response of the respiratory epithelium. Immunol Rev *173*, 27-38.

Diebold, S.S., Kaisho, T., Hemmi, H., Akira, S., and Reis e Sousa, C. (2004). Innate antiviral responses by means of TLR7-mediated recognition of single-stranded RNA. Science *303*, 1529-1531.

Diez, E., Yaraghi, Z., MacKenzie, A., and Gros, P. (2000). The neuronal apoptosis inhibitory protein (Naip) is expressed in macrophages and is modulated after phagocytosis and during intracellular infection with Legionella pneumophila. J Immunol *164*, 1470-1477.

Dohrman, A., Miyata, S., Gallup, M., Li, J.D., Chapelin, C., Coste, A., Escudier, E., Nadel, J., and Basbaum, C. (1998). Mucin gene (MUC 2 and MUC 5AC) upregulation by Gram-positive and Gram-negative bacteria. Biochim Biophys Acta *1406*, 251-259.

Dong, L.W., Kong, X.N., Yan, H.X., Yu, L.X., Chen, L., Yang, W., Liu, Q., Huang, D.D., Wu, M.C., and Wang, H.Y. (2008). Signal regulatory protein alpha negatively regulates both TLR3 and cytoplasmic pathways in type I interferon induction. Mol Immunol *45*, 3025-3035.

Doz, E., Noulin, N., Boichot, E., Guenon, I., Fick, L., Le Bert, M., Lagente, V., Ryffel, B., Schnyder, B., Quesniaux, V.F., *et al.* (2008). Cigarette smoke-induced pulmonary inflammation is TLR4/MyD88 and IL-1R1/MyD88 signaling dependent. J Immunol *180*, 1169-1178.

Duits, L.A., Nibbering, P.H., van Strijen, E., Vos, J.B., Mannesse-Lazeroms, S.P., van Sterkenburg, M.A., and Hiemstra, P.S. (2003). Rhinovirus increases human beta-defensin-2 and -3 mRNA expression in cultured bronchial epithelial cells. FEMS Immunol Med Microbiol *38*, 59-64.

Eddleston, J., Lee, R.U., Doerner, A.M., Herschbach, J., and Zuraw, B.L. (2011). Cigarette smoke decreases innate responses of epithelial cells to rhinovirus infection. Am J Respir Cell Mol Biol *44*, 118-126.

Ellison, R.T., 3rd, and Giehl, T.J. (1991). Killing of gram-negative bacteria by lactoferrin and lysozyme. J Clin Invest *88*, 1080-1091.

Franchi, L., Amer, A., Body-Malapel, M., Kanneganti, T.D., Ozoren, N., Jagirdar, R., Inohara, N., Vandenabeele, P., Bertin, J., Coyle, A., *et al.* (2006). Cytosolic flagellin requires Ipaf for activation of caspase-1 and interleukin 1beta in salmonella-infected macrophages. Nat Immunol *7*, 576-582.

Fritz, J.H., Ferrero, R.L., Philpott, D.J., and Girardin, S.E. (2006). Nod-like proteins in immunity, inflammation and disease. Nat Immunol *7*, 1250-1257.

Fritz, J.H., Girardin, S.E., Fitting, C., Werts, C., Mengin-Lecreulx, D., Caroff, M., Cavaillon, J.M., Philpott, D.J., and Adib-Conquy, M. (2005). Synergistic stimulation of human monocytes and dendritic cells by Toll-like receptor 4 and NOD1- and NOD2-activating agonists. Eur J Immunol *35*, 2459-2470.

Frutuoso, M.S., Hori, J.I., Pereira, M.S., Junior, D.S., Sonego, F., Kobayashi, K.S., Flavell, R.A., Cunha, F.Q., and Zamboni, D.S. (2010). The pattern recognition receptors Nod1 and Nod2 account for neutrophil recruitment to the lungs of mice infected with Legionella pneumophila. Microbes Infect *12*, 819-827.

Gangl, K., Reininger, R., Bernhard, D., Campana, R., Pree, I., Reisinger, J., Kneidinger, M., Kundi, M., Dolznig, H., Thurnher, D., *et al.* (2009). Cigarette smoke facilitates allergen penetration across respiratory epithelium. Allergy *64*, 398-405.

Ganz, T. (2002). Antimicrobial polypeptides in host defense of the respiratory tract. J Clin Invest *109*, 693-697.

Ganz, T. (2003). Defensins: antimicrobial peptides of innate immunity. Nat Rev Immunol *3*, 710-720.

Gensch, E., Gallup, M., Sucher, A., Li, D., Gebremichael, A., Lemjabbar, H., Mengistab, A., Dasari, V., Hotchkiss, J., Harkema, J., *et al.* (2004). Tobacco smoke control of mucin production in lung cells requires oxygen radicals AP-1 and JNK. J Biol Chem *279*, 39085-39093.

Gern, J.E., French, D.A., Grindle, K.A., Brockman-Schneider, R.A., Konno, S., and Busse, W.W. (2003). Double-stranded RNA induces the synthesis of specific chemokines by bronchial epithelial cells. Am J Respir Cell Mol Biol *28*, 731-737.

Girardin, S.E., Boneca, I.G., Carneiro, L.A., Antignac, A., Jehanno, M., Viala, J., Tedin, K., Taha, M.K., Labigne, A., Zahringer, U., *et al.* (2003a). Nod1 detects a unique muropeptide from gram-negative bacterial peptidoglycan. Science *300*, 1584-1587.

Girardin, S.E., Boneca, I.G., Viala, J., Chamaillard, M., Labigne, A., Thomas, G., Philpott, D.J., and Sansonetti, P.J. (2003b). Nod2 is a general sensor of peptidoglycan through muramyl dipeptide (MDP) detection. J Biol Chem *278*, 8869-8872.

Goldman, M.J., Anderson, G.M., Stolzenberg, E.D., Kari, U.P., Zasloff, M., and Wilson, J.M. (1997). Human beta-defensin-1 is a salt-sensitive antibiotic in lung that is inactivated in cystic fibrosis. Cell *88*, 553-560.

Greene, C.M., Carroll, T.P., Smith, S.G., Taggart, C.C., Devaney, J., Griffin, S., O'Neill S, J., and McElvaney, N.G. (2005). TLR-induced inflammation in cystic fibrosis and non-cystic fibrosis airway epithelial cells. J Immunol *174*, 1638-1646.

Guillot, L., Medjane, S., Le-Barillec, K., Balloy, V., Danel, C., Chignard, M., and Si-Tahar, M. (2004). Response of human pulmonary epithelial cells to lipopolysaccharide involves Toll-like receptor 4 (TLR4)-dependent signaling pathways: evidence for an intracellular compartmentalization of TLR4. J Biol Chem *279*, 2712-2718.

Hament, J.M., Kimpen, J.L., Fleer, A., and Wolfs, T.F. (1999). Respiratory viral infection predisposing for bacterial disease: a concise review. FEMS Immunol Med Microbiol *26*, 189-195.

Hammad, H., and Lambrecht, B.N. (2011). Dendritic cells and airway epithelial cells at the interface between innate and adaptive immune responses. Allergy *66*, 579-587.

Hartsock, A., and Nelson, W.J. (2008). Adherens and tight junctions: structure, function and connections to the actin cytoskeleton. Biochim Biophys Acta *1778*, 660-669.

Hasegawa, M., Fujimoto, Y., Lucas, P.C., Nakano, H., Fukase, K., Nunez, G., and Inohara, N. (2008). A critical role of RICK/RIP2 polyubiquitination in Nod-induced NF-kappaB activation. EMBO J *27*, 373-383.

Haswell, L.E., Hewitt, K., Thorne, D., Richter, A., and Gaca, M.D. (2010). Cigarette smoke total particulate matter increases mucous secreting cell numbers in vitro: a potential model of goblet cell hyperplasia. Toxicol In Vitro *24*, 981-987.

Hayashi, F., Smith, K.D., Ozinsky, A., Hawn, T.R., Yi, E.C., Goodlett, D.R., Eng, J.K., Akira, S., Underhill, D.M., and Aderem, A. (2001). The innate immune response to bacterial flagellin is mediated by Toll-like receptor 5. Nature *410*, 1099-1103.

Heil, F., Hemmi, H., Hochrein, H., Ampenberger, F., Kirschning, C., Akira, S., Lipford, G., Wagner, H., and Bauer, S. (2004). Species-specific recognition of single-stranded RNA via toll-like receptor 7 and 8. Science *303*, 1526-1529.

Hemmi, H., Takeuchi, O., Kawai, T., Kaisho, T., Sato, S., Sanjo, H., Matsumoto, M., Hoshino, K., Wagner, H., Takeda, K., *et al.* (2000). A Toll-like receptor recognizes bacterial DNA. Nature *408*, 740-745.

Herr, C., Beisswenger, C., Hess, C., Kandler, K., Suttorp, N., Welte, T., Schroeder, J.M., and Vogelmeier, C. (2009). Suppression of pulmonary innate host defence in smokers. Thorax *64*, 144-149.

Hoebe, K., Du, X., Georgel, P., Janssen, E., Tabeta, K., Kim, S.O., Goode, J., Lin, P., Mann, N., Mudd, S., *et al.* (2003). Identification of Lps2 as a key transducer of MyD88-independent TIR signalling. Nature *424*, 743-748.

Hoffmann, J.A. (2003). The immune response of Drosophila. Nature *426*, 33-38.

Hogg, J.C., and Timens, W. (2009). The pathology of chronic obstructive pulmonary disease. Annu Rev Pathol *4*, 435-459.

Honkinen, M., Lahti, E., Osterback, R., Ruuskanen, O., and Waris, M. (2011). Viruses and bacteria in sputum samples of children with community-acquired pneumonia. Clin Microbiol Infect.

Horng, T., Barton, G.M., Flavell, R.A., and Medzhitov, R. (2002). The adaptor molecule TIRAP provides signalling specificity for Toll-like receptors. Nature *420*, 329-333.

Ibrahim, H.R., Aoki, T., and Pellegrini, A. (2002). Strategies for new antimicrobial proteins and peptides: lysozyme and aprotinin as model molecules. Curr Pharm Des *8*, 671-693.

Ichinohe, T., Pang, I.K., and Iwasaki, A. (2010). Influenza virus activates inflammasomes via its intracellular M2 ion channel. Nat Immunol *11*, 404-410.

Innes, A.L., Woodruff, P.G., Ferrando, R.E., Donnelly, S., Dolganov, G.M., Lazarus, S.C., and Fahy, J.V. (2006). Epithelial mucin stores are increased in the large airways of smokers with airflow obstruction. Chest *130*, 1102-1108.

Ishizuka, S., Yamaya, M., Suzuki, T., Takahashi, H., Ida, S., Sasaki, T., Inoue, D., Sekizawa, K., Nishimura, H., and Sasaki, H. (2003). Effects of rhinovirus infection on the adherence of Streptococcus pneumoniae to cultured human airway epithelial cells. J Infect Dis *188*, 1928-1939.

Iyer, S.S., Pulskens, W.P., Sadler, J.J., Butter, L.M., Teske, G.J., Ulland, T.K., Eisenbarth, S.C., Florquin, S., Flavell, R.A., Leemans, J.C., *et al.* (2009). Necrotic cells trigger a sterile inflammatory response through the Nlrp3 inflammasome. Proc Natl Acad Sci U S A *106*, 20388-20393.

Jacquot, J., Tournier, J.M., and Puchelle, E. (1985). In vitro evidence that human airway lysozyme is cleaved and inactivated by Pseudomonas aeruginosa elastase and not by human leukocyte elastase. Infect Immun *47*, 555-560.

Jamieson, A.M., Yu, S., Annicelli, C.H., and Medzhitov, R. (2010). Influenza virus-induced glucocorticoids compromise innate host defense against a secondary bacterial infection. Cell Host Microbe *7*, 103-114.

Jansen, H.M., Sachs, A.P., and van Alphen, L. (1995). Predisposing conditions to bacterial infections in chronic obstructive pulmonary disease. Am J Respir Crit Care Med *151*, 2073-2080.

Jeong, E., and Lee, J.Y. (2011). Intrinsic and extrinsic regulation of innate immune receptors. Yonsei Med J *52*, 379-392.

Jia, H.P., Kline, J.N., Penisten, A., Apicella, M.A., Gioannini, T.L., Weiss, J., and McCray, P.B., Jr. (2004). Endotoxin responsiveness of human airway epithelia is limited by low expression of MD-2. Am J Physiol Lung Cell Mol Physiol *287*, L428-437.

Jiang, Z., Nagata, N., Molina, E., Bakaletz, L.O., Hawkins, H., and Patel, J.A. (1999). Fimbria-mediated enhanced attachment of nontypeable Haemophilus influenzae to respiratory syncytial virus-infected respiratory epithelial cells. Infect Immun *67*, 187-192.

John, G., Yildirim, A.O., Rubin, B.K., Gruenert, D.C., and Henke, M.O. (2010). TLR-4-mediated innate immunity is reduced in cystic fibrosis airway cells. Am J Respir Cell Mol Biol *42*, 424-431.

Kagan, J.C., Su, T., Horng, T., Chow, A., Akira, S., and Medzhitov, R. (2008). TRAM couples endocytosis of Toll-like receptor 4 to the induction of interferon-beta. Nat Immunol *9*, 361-368.

Kang, D.C., Gopalkrishnan, R.V., Wu, Q., Jankowsky, E., Pyle, A.M., and Fisher, P.B. (2002). mda-5: An interferon-inducible putative RNA helicase with double-stranded RNA-dependent ATPase activity and melanoma growth-suppressive properties. Proc Natl Acad Sci U S A *99*, 637-642.

Kang, M.J., Lee, C.G., Lee, J.Y., Dela Cruz, C.S., Chen, Z.J., Enelow, R., and Elias, J.A. (2008). Cigarette smoke selectively enhances viral PAMP- and virus-induced pulmonary innate immune and remodeling responses in mice. J Clin Invest *118*, 2771-2784.

Kanneganti, T.D. (2010). Central roles of NLRs and inflammasomes in viral infection. Nat Rev Immunol *10*, 688-698.

Kanneganti, T.D., Lamkanfi, M., and Nunez, G. (2007). Intracellular NOD-like receptors in host defense and disease. Immunity *27*, 549-559.

Kanneganti, T.D., Ozoren, N., Body-Malapel, M., Amer, A., Park, J.H., Franchi, L., Whitfield, J., Barchet, W., Colonna, M., Vandenabeele, P., *et al.* (2006). Bacterial RNA and small antiviral compounds activate caspase-1 through cryopyrin/Nalp3. Nature *440*, 233-236.

Kato, A., and Schleimer, R.P. (2007). Beyond inflammation: airway epithelial cells are at the interface of innate and adaptive immunity. Curr Opin Immunol *19*, 711-720.

Kato, H., Sato, S., Yoneyama, M., Yamamoto, M., Uematsu, S., Matsui, K., Tsujimura, T., Takeda, K., Fujita, T., Takeuchi, O., *et al.* (2005). Cell type-specific involvement of RIG-I in antiviral response. Immunity *23*, 19-28.

Kato, H., Takeuchi, O., Mikamo-Satoh, E., Hirai, R., Kawai, T., Matsushita, K., Hiiragi, A., Dermody, T.S., Fujita, T., and Akira, S. (2008). Length-dependent recognition of double-stranded ribonucleic acids by retinoic acid-inducible gene-I and melanoma differentiation-associated gene 5. J Exp Med *205*, 1601-1610.

Kato, H., Takeuchi, O., Sato, S., Yoneyama, M., Yamamoto, M., Matsui, K., Uematsu, S., Jung, A., Kawai, T., Ishii, K.J., *et al.* (2006). Differential roles of MDA5 and RIG-I helicases in the recognition of RNA viruses. Nature *441*, 101-105.

Kawai, T., Adachi, O., Ogawa, T., Takeda, K., and Akira, S. (1999). Unresponsiveness of MyD88-deficient mice to endotoxin. Immunity *11*, 115-122.

Kawai, T., and Akira, S. (2008). Toll-like receptor and RIG-I-like receptor signaling. Ann N Y Acad Sci *1143*, 1-20.

Kawai, T., and Akira, S. (2009). The roles of TLRs, RLRs and NLRs in pathogen recognition. Int Immunol *21*, 317-337.

Kawai, T., Takahashi, K., Sato, S., Coban, C., Kumar, H., Kato, H., Ishii, K.J., Takeuchi, O., and Akira, S. (2005). IPS-1, an adaptor triggering RIG-I- and Mda5-mediated type I interferon induction. Nat Immunol *6*, 981-988.

Khan, E.M., Lanir, R., Danielson, A.R., and Goldkorn, T. (2008). Epidermal growth factor receptor exposed to cigarette smoke is aberrantly activated and undergoes perinuclear trafficking. FASEB J *22*, 910-917.

Knowles, M.R., and Boucher, R.C. (2002). Mucus clearance as a primary innate defense mechanism for mammalian airways. J Clin Invest *109*, 571-577.

Koch, S., and Nusrat, A. (2009). Dynamic regulation of epithelial cell fate and barrier function by intercellular junctions. Ann N Y Acad Sci *1165*, 220-227.

Kohri, K., Ueki, I.F., Shim, J.J., Burgel, P.R., Oh, Y.M., Tam, D.C., Dao-Pick, T., and Nadel, J.A. (2002). Pseudomonas aeruginosa induces MUC5AC production via epidermal growth factor receptor. Eur Respir J *20*, 1263-1270.

Komori, M., Inoue, H., Matsumoto, K., Koto, H., Fukuyama, S., Aizawa, H., and Hara, N. (2001). PAF mediates cigarette smoke-induced goblet cell metaplasia in guinea pig airways. Am J Physiol Lung Cell Mol Physiol *280*, L436-441.

Kota, S., Sabbah, A., Chang, T.H., Harnack, R., Xiang, Y., Meng, X., and Bose, S. (2008). Role of human beta-defensin-2 during tumor necrosis factor-alpha/NF-kappaB-mediated innate antiviral response against human respiratory syncytial virus. J Biol Chem *283*, 22417-22429.

Kulkarni, R., Rampersaud, R., Aguilar, J.L., Randis, T.M., Kreindler, J.L., and Ratner, A.J. (2010). Cigarette smoke inhibits airway epithelial cell innate immune responses to bacteria. Infect Immun *78*, 2146-2152.

Kurt-Jones, E.A., Popova, L., Kwinn, L., Haynes, L.M., Jones, L.P., Tripp, R.A., Walsh, E.E., Freeman, M.W., Golenbock, D.T., Anderson, L.J., *et al.* (2000). Pattern recognition receptors TLR4 and CD14 mediate response to respiratory syncytial virus. Nat Immunol *1*, 398-401.

Lachowicz-Scroggins, M.E., Boushey, H.A., Finkbeiner, W.E., and Widdicombe, J.H. (2010). Interleukin-13-induced mucous metaplasia increases susceptibility of human airway epithelium to rhinovirus infection. Am J Respir Cell Mol Biol *43*, 652-661.

Landry, R.M., An, D., Hupp, J.T., Singh, P.K., and Parsek, M.R. (2006). Mucin-Pseudomonas aeruginosa interactions promote biofilm formation and antibiotic resistance. Mol Microbiol *59*, 142-151.

Lappalainen, U., Whitsett, J.A., Wert, S.E., Tichelaar, J.W., and Bry, K. (2005). Interleukin-1beta causes pulmonary inflammation, emphysema, and airway remodeling in the adult murine lung. Am J Respir Cell Mol Biol *32*, 311-318.

Laube, D.M., Yim, S., Ryan, L.K., Kisich, K.O., and Diamond, G. (2006). Antimicrobial peptides in the airway. Curr Top Microbiol Immunol *306*, 153-182.

Lemjabbar, H., Li, D., Gallup, M., Sidhu, S., Drori, E., and Basbaum, C. (2003). Tobacco smoke-induced lung cell proliferation mediated by tumor necrosis factor alpha-converting enzyme and amphiregulin. J Biol Chem *278*, 26202-26207.

Li, C., Zienkiewicz, J., and Hawiger, J. (2005). Interactive sites in the MyD88 Toll/interleukin (IL) 1 receptor domain responsible for coupling to the IL1beta signaling pathway. J Biol Chem *280*, 26152-26159.

Li, J.D., Dohrman, A.F., Gallup, M., Miyata, S., Gum, J.R., Kim, Y.S., Nadel, J.A., Prince, A., and Basbaum, C.B. (1997). Transcriptional activation of mucin by Pseudomonas aeruginosa lipopolysaccharide in the pathogenesis of cystic fibrosis lung disease. Proc Natl Acad Sci U S A *94*, 967-972.

Liu, P., Jamaluddin, M., Li, K., Garofalo, R.P., Casola, A., and Brasier, A.R. (2007). Retinoic acid-inducible gene I mediates early antiviral response and Toll-like receptor 3 expression in respiratory syncytial virus-infected airway epithelial cells. J Virol *81*, 1401-1411.

Livraghi, A., and Randell, S.H. (2007). Cystic fibrosis and other respiratory diseases of impaired mucus clearance. Toxicol Pathol *35*, 116-129.

MacRedmond, R.E., Greene, C.M., Dorscheid, D.R., McElvaney, N.G., and O'Neill, S.J. (2007). Epithelial expression of TLR4 is modulated in COPD and by steroids, salmeterol and cigarette smoke. Respir Res *8*, 84.

Mariathasan, S., Weiss, D.S., Newton, K., McBride, J., O'Rourke, K., Roose-Girma, M., Lee, W.P., Weinrauch, Y., Monack, D.M., and Dixit, V.M. (2006). Cryopyrin activates the inflammasome in response to toxins and ATP. Nature *440*, 228-232.

Martinon, F., Agostini, L., Meylan, E., and Tschopp, J. (2004). Identification of bacterial muramyl dipeptide as activator of the NALP3/cryopyrin inflammasome. Curr Biol *14*, 1929-1934.

Martinon, F., Burns, K., and Tschopp, J. (2002). The inflammasome: a molecular platform triggering activation of inflammatory caspases and processing of proIL-beta. Mol Cell *10*, 417-426.

Martinon, F., Petrilli, V., Mayor, A., Tardivel, A., and Tschopp, J. (2006). Gout-associated uric acid crystals activate the NALP3 inflammasome. Nature *440*, 237-241.

Masui, T., Lechner, J.F., Yoakum, G.H., Willey, J.C., and Harris, C.C. (1986a). Growth and differentiation of normal and transformed human bronchial epithelial cells. J Cell Physiol Suppl *4*, 73-81.

Masui, T., Wakefield, L.M., Lechner, J.F., LaVeck, M.A., Sporn, M.B., and Harris, C.C. (1986b). Type beta transforming growth factor is the primary differentiation-inducing serum factor for normal human bronchial epithelial cells. Proc Natl Acad Sci U S A *83*, 2438-2442.

Matrosovich, M., and Klenk, H.D. (2003). Natural and synthetic sialic acid-containing inhibitors of influenza virus receptor binding. Rev Med Virol *13*, 85-97.

Mayer, A.K., Muehmer, M., Mages, J., Gueinzius, K., Hess, C., Heeg, K., Bals, R., Lang, R., and Dalpke, A.H. (2007). Differential recognition of TLR-dependent microbial ligands in human bronchial epithelial cells. J Immunol *178*, 3134-3142.

Mazieres, J., He, B., You, L., Xu, Z., and Jablons, D.M. (2005). Wnt signaling in lung cancer. Cancer Lett *222*, 1-10.

McCray, P.B., Jr., and Bentley, L. (1997). Human airway epithelia express a beta-defensin. Am J Respir Cell Mol Biol *16*, 343-349.

McCullers, J.A. (2006). Insights into the interaction between influenza virus and pneumococcus. Clin Microbiol Rev *19*, 571-582.

McElvaney, N.G., Nakamura, H., Birrer, P., Hebert, C.A., Wong, W.L., Alphonso, M., Baker, J.B., Catalano, M.A., and Crystal, R.G. (1992). Modulation of airway inflammation in cystic fibrosis. In vivo suppression of interleukin-8 levels on the respiratory epithelial surface by aerosolization of recombinant secretory leukoprotease inhibitor. J Clin Invest *90*, 1296-1301.

McGillivary, G., Mason, K.M., Jurcisek, J.A., Peeples, M.E., and Bakaletz, L.O. (2009). Respiratory syncytial virus-induced dysregulation of expression of a mucosal beta-defensin augments colonization of the upper airway by non-typeable Haemophilus influenzae. Cell Microbiol *11*, 1399-1408.

Mebratu, Y.A., Schwalm, K., Smith, K.R., Schuyler, M., and Tesfaigzi, Y. (2011). Cigarette smoke suppresses Bik to cause epithelial cell hyperplasia and mucous cell metaplasia. Am J Respir Crit Care Med *183*, 1531-1538.

Medzhitov, R. (2001). Toll-like receptors and innate immunity. Nat Rev Immunol *1*, 135-145.

Medzhitov, R., and Janeway, C.A., Jr. (1997). Innate immunity: impact on the adaptive immune response. Curr Opin Immunol *9*, 4-9.

Mehta, H., Nazzal, K., and Sadikot, R.T. (2008). Cigarette smoking and innate immunity. Inflamm Res *57*, 497-503.

Meixenberger, K., Pache, F., Eitel, J., Schmeck, B., Hippenstiel, S., Slevogt, H., N'Guessan, P., Witzenrath, M., Netea, M.G., Chakraborty, T., *et al.* (2010). Listeria monocytogenes-infected human peripheral blood mononuclear cells produce IL-1beta, depending on listeriolysin O and NLRP3. J Immunol *184*, 922-930.

Meylan, E., Curran, J., Hofmann, K., Moradpour, D., Binder, M., Bartenschlager, R., and Tschopp, J. (2005). Cardif is an adaptor protein in the RIG-I antiviral pathway and is targeted by hepatitis C virus. Nature *437*, 1167-1172.

Meylan, E., and Tschopp, J. (2006). Toll-like receptors and RNA helicases: two parallel ways to trigger antiviral responses. Mol Cell *22*, 561-569.

Miao, E.A., Alpuche-Aranda, C.M., Dors, M., Clark, A.E., Bader, M.W., Miller, S.I., and Aderem, A. (2006). Cytoplasmic flagellin activates caspase-1 and secretion of interleukin 1beta via Ipaf. Nat Immunol *7*, 569-575.

Modestou, M.A., Manzel, L.J., El-Mahdy, S., and Look, D.C. (2010). Inhibition of IFN-gamma-dependent antiviral airway epithelial defense by cigarette smoke. Respir Res *11*, 64.

Moore, C.B., Bergstralh, D.T., Duncan, J.A., Lei, Y., Morrison, T.E., Zimmermann, A.G., Accavitti-Loper, M.A., Madden, V.J., Sun, L., Ye, Z., *et al.* (2008). NLRX1 is a regulator of mitochondrial antiviral immunity. Nature *451*, 573-577.

Moskwa, P., Lorentzen, D., Excoffon, K.J., Zabner, J., McCray, P.B., Jr., Nauseef, W.M., Dupuy, C., and Banfi, B. (2007). A novel host defense system of airways is defective in cystic fibrosis. Am J Respir Crit Care Med *175*, 174-183.

Mukaida, N., Mahe, Y., and Matsushima, K. (1990). Cooperative interaction of nuclear factor-kappa B- and cis-regulatory enhancer binding protein-like factor binding elements in activating the interleukin-8 gene by pro-inflammatory cytokines. J Biol Chem *265*, 21128-21133.

Murphy, T.F. (2000). Haemophilus influenzae in chronic bronchitis. Semin Respir Infect *15*, 41-51.

Murphy, T.F., Brauer, A.L., Eschberger, K., Lobbins, P., Grove, L., Cai, X., and Sethi, S. (2008). Pseudomonas aeruginosa in chronic obstructive pulmonary disease. Am J Respir Crit Care Med *177*, 853-860.

Murphy, T.F., Brauer, A.L., Sethi, S., Kilian, M., Cai, X., and Lesse, A.J. (2007). Haemophilus haemolyticus: a human respiratory tract commensal to be distinguished from Haemophilus influenzae. J Infect Dis *195*, 81-89.

Muruve, D.A., Petrilli, V., Zaiss, A.K., White, L.R., Clark, S.A., Ross, P.J., Parks, R.J., and Tschopp, J. (2008). The inflammasome recognizes cytosolic microbial and host DNA and triggers an innate immune response. Nature *452*, 103-107.

O'Donnell, R.A., Richter, A., Ward, J., Angco, G., Mehta, A., Rousseau, K., Swallow, D.M., Holgate, S.T., Djukanovic, R., Davies, D.E., *et al.* (2004). Expression of ErbB receptors and mucins in the airways of long term current smokers. Thorax *59*, 1032-1040.

Oliver, B.G., Lim, S., Wark, P., Laza-Stanca, V., King, N., Black, J.L., Burgess, J.K., Roth, M., and Johnston, S.L. (2008). Rhinovirus exposure impairs immune responses to bacterial products in human alveolar macrophages. Thorax *63*, 519-525.

Olivera, D.S., Boggs, S.E., Beenhouwer, C., Aden, J., and Knall, C. (2007). Cellular mechanisms of mainstream cigarette smoke-induced lung epithelial tight junction permeability changes in vitro. Inhal Toxicol *19*, 13-22.

Ong, E.L., Ellis, M.E., Webb, A.K., Neal, K.R., Dodd, M., Caul, E.O., and Burgess, S. (1989). Infective respiratory exacerbations in young adults with cystic fibrosis: role of viruses and atypical microorganisms. Thorax *44*, 739-742.

Opitz, B., Puschel, A., Schmeck, B., Hocke, A.C., Rosseau, S., Hammerschmidt, S., Schumann, R.R., Suttorp, N., and Hippenstiel, S. (2004). Nucleotide-binding oligomerization domain proteins are innate immune receptors for internalized Streptococcus pneumoniae. J Biol Chem *279*, 36426-36432.

Pace, E., Ferraro, M., Siena, L., Melis, M., Montalbano, A.M., Johnson, M., Bonsignore, M.R., Bonsignore, G., and Gjomarkaj, M. (2008). Cigarette smoke increases Toll-like receptor 4 and modifies lipopolysaccharide-mediated responses in airway epithelial cells. Immunology *124*, 401-411.

Pace, E., Giarratano, A., Ferraro, M., Bruno, A., Siena, L., Mangione, S., Johnson, M., and Gjomarkaj, M. (2011). TLR4 upregulation underpins airway neutrophilia in smokers with chronic obstructive pulmonary disease and acute respiratory failure. Hum Immunol *72*, 54-62.

Papi, A., Bellettato, C.M., Braccioni, F., Romagnoli, M., Casolari, P., Caramori, G., Fabbri, L.M., and Johnston, S.L. (2006). Infections and airway inflammation in chronic obstructive pulmonary disease severe exacerbations. Am J Respir Crit Care Med *173*, 1114-1121.

Parameswaran, G.I., Sethi, S., and Murphy, T.F. (2011). Effects of Bacterial Infection on Airway Antimicrobial Peptides and Proteins in Chronic Obstructive Pulmonary Disease. Chest.

Parameswaran, G.I., Wrona, C.T., Murphy, T.F., and Sethi, S. (2009). Moraxella catarrhalis acquisition, airway inflammation and protease-antiprotease balance in chronic obstructive pulmonary disease. BMC Infect Dis *9*, 178.

Passariello, C., Schippa, S., Conti, C., Russo, P., Poggiali, F., Garaci, E., and Palamara, A.T. (2006). Rhinoviruses promote internalisation of Staphylococcus aureus into non-fully permissive cultured pneumocytes. Microbes Infect *8*, 758-766.

Piao, W., Song, C., Chen, H., Diaz, M.A., Wahl, L.M., Fitzgerald, K.A., Li, L., and Medvedev, A.E. (2009). Endotoxin tolerance dysregulates MyD88- and Toll/IL-1R domain-containing adapter inducing IFN-beta-dependent pathways and increases expression of negative regulators of TLR signaling. J Leukoc Biol *86*, 863-875.

Platz, J., Beisswenger, C., Dalpke, A., Koczulla, R., Pinkenburg, O., Vogelmeier, C., and Bals, R. (2004). Microbial DNA induces a host defense reaction of human respiratory epithelial cells. J Immunol *173*, 1219-1223.

Plotkowski, M.C., Bajolet-Laudinat, O., and Puchelle, E. (1993). Cellular and molecular mechanisms of bacterial adhesion to respiratory mucosa. Eur Respir J *6*, 903-916.

Pohl, C., Hermanns, M.I., Uboldi, C., Bock, M., Fuchs, S., Dei-Anang, J., Mayer, E., Kehe, K., Kummer, W., and Kirkpatrick, C.J. (2009). Barrier functions and paracellular integrity in human cell culture models of the proximal respiratory unit. Eur J Pharm Biopharm *72*, 339-349.

Poltorak, A., He, X., Smirnova, I., Liu, M.Y., Van Huffel, C., Du, X., Birdwell, D., Alejos, E., Silva, M., Galanos, C., *et al.* (1998). Defective LPS signaling in C3H/HeJ and C57BL/10ScCr mice: mutations in Tlr4 gene. Science *282*, 2085-2088.

Ramsey, B.W., Gore, E.J., Smith, A.L., Cooney, M.K., Redding, G.J., and Foy, H. (1989). The effect of respiratory viral infections on patients with cystic fibrosis. Am J Dis Child *143*, 662-668.

Rose, M.C., Nickola, T.J., and Voynow, J.A. (2001). Airway mucus obstruction: mucin glycoproteins, MUC gene regulation and goblet cell hyperplasia. Am J Respir Cell Mol Biol *25*, 533-537.

Rose, M.C., and Voynow, J.A. (2006). Respiratory tract mucin genes and mucin glycoproteins in health and disease. Physiol Rev *86*, 245-278.

Ryan, P.A., Pancholi, V., and Fischetti, V.A. (2001). Group A streptococci bind to mucin and human pharyngeal cells through sialic acid-containing receptors. Infect Immun *69*, 7402-7412.

Sabbah, A., Chang, T.H., Harnack, R., Frohlich, V., Tominaga, K., Dube, P.H., Xiang, Y., and Bose, S. (2009). Activation of innate immune antiviral responses by Nod2. Nat Immunol *10*, 1073-1080.

Sajjan, S.U., and Forstner, J.F. (1992). Identification of the mucin-binding adhesin of Pseudomonas cepacia isolated from patients with cystic fibrosis. Infect Immun *60*, 1434-1440.

Sajjan, U., Ganesan, S., Comstock, A.T., Shim, J., Wang, Q., Nagarkar, D.R., Zhao, Y., Goldsmith, A.M., Sonstein, J., Linn, M.J., *et al.* (2009). Elastase- and LPS-exposed mice display altered responses to rhinovirus infection. Am J Physiol Lung Cell Mol Physiol *297*, L931-944.

Sajjan, U., Wang, Q., Zhao, Y., Gruenert, D.C., and Hershenson, M.B. (2008). Rhinovirus disrupts the barrier function of polarized airway epithelial cells. Am J Respir Crit Care Med *178*, 1271-1281.

Sajjan, U.S., Corey, M., Karmali, M.A., and Forstner, J.F. (1992). Binding of Pseudomonas cepacia to normal human intestinal mucin and respiratory mucin from patients with cystic fibrosis. J Clin Invest *89*, 648-656.

Sajjan, U.S., Jia, Y., Newcomb, D.C., Bentley, J.K., Lukacs, N.W., LiPuma, J.J., and Hershenson, M.B. (2006). H. influenzae potentiates airway epithelial cell responses to rhinovirus by increasing ICAM-1 and TLR3 expression. FASEB J *20*, 2121-2123.

Sapey, E., Ahmad, A., Bayley, D., Newbold, P., Snell, N., Rugman, P., and Stockley, R.A. (2009). Imbalances between interleukin-1 and tumor necrosis factor agonists and antagonists in stable COPD. J Clin Immunol *29*, 508-516.

Sarkar, S.N., Peters, K.L., Elco, C.P., Sakamoto, S., Pal, S., and Sen, G.C. (2004). Novel roles of TLR3 tyrosine phosphorylation and PI3 kinase in double-stranded RNA signaling. Nat Struct Mol Biol *11*, 1060-1067.

Savitski, A.N., Mesaros, C., Blair, I.A., Cohen, N.A., and Kreindler, J.L. (2009). Secondhand smoke inhibits both Cl- and K+ conductances in normal human bronchial epithelial cells. Respir Res *10*, 120.

Schneeberger, E.E., and Lynch, R.D. (2004). The tight junction: a multifunctional complex. Am J Physiol Cell Physiol *286*, C1213-1228.

Schneider, D., Ganesan, S., Comstock, A.T., Meldrum, C.A., Mahidhara, R., Goldsmith, A.M., Curtis, J.L., Martinez, F.J., Hershenson, M.B., and Sajjan, U. (2010). Increased cytokine response of rhinovirus-infected airway epithelial cells in chronic obstructive pulmonary disease. Am J Respir Crit Care Med *182*, 332-340.

Schwandner, R., Dziarski, R., Wesche, H., Rothe, M., and Kirschning, C.J. (1999). Peptidoglycan- and lipoteichoic acid-induced cell activation is mediated by toll-like receptor 2. J Biol Chem *274*, 17406-17409.

Seki, M., Higashiyama, Y., Tomono, K., Yanagihara, K., Ohno, H., Kaneko, Y., Izumikawa, K., Miyazaki, Y., Hirakata, Y., Mizuta, Y., *et al.* (2004). Acute infection with influenza virus enhances susceptibility to fatal pneumonia following Streptococcus pneumoniae infection in mice with chronic pulmonary colonization with Pseudomonas aeruginosa. Clin Exp Immunol *137*, 35-40.

Serikov, V.B., Leutenegger, C., Krutilina, R., Kropotov, A., Pleskach, N., Suh, J.H., and Tomilin, N.V. (2006). Cigarette smoke extract inhibits expression of peroxiredoxin V and increases airway epithelial permeability. Inhal Toxicol *18*, 79-92.

Seth, R.B., Sun, L., Ea, C.K., and Chen, Z.J. (2005). Identification and characterization of MAVS, a mitochondrial antiviral signaling protein that activates NF-kappaB and IRF 3. Cell *122*, 669-682.

Sethi, S. (2000). Bacterial infection and the pathogenesis of COPD. Chest *117*, 286S-291S.

Sethi, S., Maloney, J., Grove, L., Wrona, C., and Berenson, C.S. (2006). Airway inflammation and bronchial bacterial colonization in chronic obstructive pulmonary disease. Am J Respir Crit Care Med *173*, 991-998.

Sethi, S., and Murphy, T.F. (2008). Infection in the pathogenesis and course of chronic obstructive pulmonary disease. N Engl J Med *359*, 2355-2365.

Sha, Q., Truong-Tran, A.Q., Plitt, J.R., Beck, L.A., and Schleimer, R.P. (2004). Activation of airway epithelial cells by toll-like receptor agonists. Am J Respir Cell Mol Biol *31*, 358-364.

Shao, M.X., Nakanaga, T., and Nadel, J.A. (2004). Cigarette smoke induces MUC5AC mucin overproduction via tumor necrosis factor-alpha-converting enzyme in human airway epithelial (NCI-H292) cells. American journal of physiology *287*, L420-427.

Shaykhiev, R., Otaki, F., Bonsu, P., Dang, D.T., Teater, M., Strulovici-Barel, Y., Salit, J., Harvey, B.G., and Crystal, R.G. (2011). Cigarette smoking reprograms apical junctional complex molecular architecture in the human airway epithelium in vivo. Cell Mol Life Sci *68*, 877-892.

Shimada, K., Chen, S., Dempsey, P.W., Sorrentino, R., Alsabeh, R., Slepenkin, A.V., Peterson, E., Doherty, T.M., Underhill, D., Crother, T.R., *et al.* (2009). The NOD/RIP2 pathway is essential for host defenses against Chlamydophila pneumoniae lung infection. PLoS Pathog *5*, e1000379.

Shin, K., Fogg, V.C., and Margolis, B. (2006). Tight junctions and cell polarity. Annu Rev Cell Dev Biol *22*, 207-235.

Simet, S.M., Sisson, J.H., Pavlik, J.A., Devasure, J.M., Boyer, C., Liu, X., Kawasaki, S., Sharp, J.G., Rennard, S.I., and Wyatt, T.A. (2010). Long-term cigarette smoke exposure in a mouse model of ciliated epithelial cell function. Am J Respir Cell Mol Biol *43*, 635-640.

Singh, P.K., Jia, H.P., Wiles, K., Hesselberth, J., Liu, L., Conway, B.A., Greenberg, E.P., Valore, E.V., Welsh, M.J., Ganz, T., *et al.* (1998). Production of beta-defensins by human airway epithelia. Proc Natl Acad Sci U S A *95*, 14961-14966.

Sly, L.M., Hamilton, M.J., Kuroda, E., Ho, V.W., Antignano, F.L., Omeis, S.L., van Netten-Thomas, C.J., Wong, D., Brugger, H.K., Williams, O., *et al.* (2009). SHIP prevents lipopolysaccharide from triggering an antiviral response in mice. Blood *113*, 2945-2954.

Soong, G., Reddy, B., Sokol, S., Adamo, R., and Prince, A. (2004). TLR2 is mobilized into an apical lipid raft receptor complex to signal infection in airway epithelial cells. J Clin Invest *113*, 1482-1489.

Sun, K., and Metzger, D.W. (2008). Inhibition of pulmonary antibacterial defense by interferon-gamma during recovery from influenza infection. Nat Med *14*, 558-564.

Sun, Q., Sun, L., Liu, H.H., Chen, X., Seth, R.B., Forman, J., and Chen, Z.J. (2006). The specific and essential role of MAVS in antiviral innate immune responses. Immunity *24*, 633-642.

Sykes, A., Mallia, P., and Johnston, S.L. (2007). Diagnosis of pathogens in exacerbations of chronic obstructive pulmonary disease. Proc Am Thorac Soc *4*, 642-646.

Taggart, C.C., Lowe, G.J., Greene, C.M., Mulgrew, A.T., O'Neill, S.J., Levine, R.L., and McElvaney, N.G. (2001). Cathepsin B, L, and S cleave and inactivate secretory leucoprotease inhibitor. J Biol Chem *276*, 33345-33352.

Takeuchi, O., Kawai, T., Muhlradt, P.F., Morr, M., Radolf, J.D., Zychlinsky, A., Takeda, K., and Akira, S. (2001). Discrimination of bacterial lipoproteins by Toll-like receptor 6. Int Immunol *13*, 933-940.

Takeuchi, O., Sato, S., Horiuchi, T., Hoshino, K., Takeda, K., Dong, Z., Modlin, R.L., and Akira, S. (2002). Cutting edge: role of Toll-like receptor 1 in mediating immune response to microbial lipoproteins. J Immunol *169*, 10-14.

Tamashiro, E., Xiong, G., Anselmo-Lima, W.T., Kreindler, J.L., Palmer, J.N., and Cohen, N.A. (2009). Cigarette smoke exposure impairs respiratory epithelial ciliogenesis. Am J Rhinol Allergy *23*, 117-122.

Tattoli, I., Carneiro, L.A., Jehanno, M., Magalhaes, J.G., Shu, Y., Philpott, D.J., Arnoult, D., and Girardin, S.E. (2008). NLRX1 is a mitochondrial NOD-like receptor that amplifies NF-kappaB and JNK pathways by inducing reactive oxygen species production. EMBO Rep *9*, 293-300.

Taylor, D.C., Cripps, A.W., and Clancy, R.L. (1995). A possible role for lysozyme in determining acute exacerbation in chronic bronchitis. Clin Exp Immunol *102*, 406-416.

Thomas, P.G., Dash, P., Aldridge, J.R., Jr., Ellebedy, A.H., Reynolds, C., Funk, A.J., Martin, W.J., Lamkanfi, M., Webby, R.J., Boyd, K.L., *et al.* (2009). The intracellular sensor NLRP3 mediates key innate and healing responses to influenza A virus via the regulation of caspase-1. Immunity *30*, 566-575.

Thornton, D.J., Rousseau, K., and McGuckin, M.A. (2008). Structure and function of the polymeric mucins in airways mucus. Annu Rev Physiol *70*, 459-486.

Tian, D., Zhu, M., Li, J., Ma, Y., and Wu, R. (2009). Cigarette smoke extract induces activation of beta-catenin/TCF signaling through inhibiting GSK3beta in human alveolar epithelial cell line. Toxicol Lett *187*, 58-62.

Travassos, L.H., Carneiro, L.A., Girardin, S.E., Boneca, I.G., Lemos, R., Bozza, M.T., Domingues, R.C., Coyle, A.J., Bertin, J., Philpott, D.J., *et al.* (2005). Nod1 participates in the innate immune response to Pseudomonas aeruginosa. J Biol Chem *280*, 36714-36718.

Tsoumakidou, M., Bouloukaki, I., Thimaki, K., Tzanakis, N., and Siafakas, N.M. (2010). Innate immunity proteins in chronic obstructive pulmonary disease and idiopathic pulmonary fibrosis. Exp Lung Res *36*, 373-380.

Ueno, K., Koga, T., Kato, K., Golenbock, D.T., Gendler, S.J., Kai, H., and Kim, K.C. (2008). MUC1 mucin is a negative regulator of toll-like receptor signaling. Am J Respir Cell Mol Biol *38*, 263-268.

Urban, T.A., Griffith, A., Torok, A.M., Smolkin, M.E., Burns, J.L., and Goldberg, J.B. (2004). Contribution of Burkholderia cenocepacia flagella to infectivity and inflammation. Infect Immun *72*, 5126-5134.

van der Strate, B.W., Beljaars, L., Molema, G., Harmsen, M.C., and Meijer, D.K. (2001). Antiviral activities of lactoferrin. Antiviral Res *52*, 225-239.

Van Ewijk, B.E., Wolfs, T.F., Aerts, P.C., Van Kessel, K.P., Fleer, A., Kimpen, J.L., and Van der Ent, C.K. (2007). RSV mediates Pseudomonas aeruginosa binding to cystic fibrosis and normal epithelial cells. Pediatr Res *61*, 398-403.

Vinzing, M., Eitel, J., Lippmann, J., Hocke, A.C., Zahlten, J., Slevogt, H., N'Guessan P, D., Gunther, S., Schmeck, B., Hippenstiel, S., *et al.* (2008). NAIP and Ipaf control Legionella pneumophila replication in human cells. J Immunol *180*, 6808-6815.

Voynow, J.A., Gendler, S.J., and Rose, M.C. (2006). Regulation of mucin genes in chronic inflammatory airway diseases. Am J Respir Cell Mol Biol *34*, 661-665.

Walters, R.W., Pilewski, J.M., Chiorini, J.A., and Zabner, J. (2002). Secreted and transmembrane mucins inhibit gene transfer with AAV4 more efficiently than AAV5. J Biol Chem *277*, 23709-23713.

Wanderer, A.A. (2008). Interleukin-1beta targeted therapy in severe persistent asthma (SPA) and chronic obstructive pulmonary disease (COPD): proposed similarities between biphasic pathobiology of SPA/COPD and ischemia-reperfusion injury. Isr Med Assoc J *10*, 837-842.

Wang, A., Yokosaki, Y., Ferrando, R., Balmes, J., and Sheppard, D. (1996). Differential regulation of airway epithelial integrins by growth factors. Am J Respir Cell Mol Biol *15*, 664-672.

Wang, Q., Miller, D.J., Bowman, E.R., Nagarkar, D.R., Schneider, D., Zhao, Y., Linn, M.J., Goldsmith, A.M., Bentley, J.K., Sajjan, U.S., *et al.* (2011). MDA5 and TLR3 initiate pro-inflammatory signaling pathways leading to rhinovirus-induced airways inflammation and hyperresponsiveness. PLoS Pathog *7*, e1002070.

Wang, Q., Nagarkar, D.R., Bowman, E.R., Schneider, D., Gosangi, B., Lei, J., Zhao, Y., McHenry, C.L., Burgens, R.V., Miller, D.J., *et al.* (2009). Role of double-stranded RNA pattern recognition receptors in rhinovirus-induced airway epithelial cell responses. J Immunol *183*, 6989-6997.

Wat, D., Gelder, C., Hibbitts, S., Cafferty, F., Bowler, I., Pierrepoint, M., Evans, R., and Doull, I. (2008). The role of respiratory viruses in cystic fibrosis. J Cyst Fibros *7*, 320-328.

Wilkinson, T.M., Hurst, J.R., Perera, W.R., Wilks, M., Donaldson, G.C., and Wedzicha, J.A. (2006). Effect of interactions between lower airway bacterial and rhinoviral infection in exacerbations of COPD. Chest *129*, 317-324.

Wilson, R. (2000). Evidence of bacterial infection in acute exacerbations of chronic bronchitis. Semin Respir Infect *15*, 208-215.

Wu, W., Patel, K.B., Booth, J.L., Zhang, W., and Metcalf, J.P. (2011). Cigarette smoke extract suppresses the RIG-I-initiated innate immune response to influenza virus in the human lung. Am J Physiol Lung Cell Mol Physiol *300*, L821-830.

Xing, Z., Harper, R., Anunciacion, J., Yang, Z., Gao, W., Qu, B., Guan, Y., and Cardona, C.J. (2011). Host immune and apoptotic responses to avian influenza virus H9N2 in human tracheobronchial epithelial cells. Am J Respir Cell Mol Biol *44*, 24-33.

Xu, L.G., Wang, Y.Y., Han, K.J., Li, L.Y., Zhai, Z., and Shu, H.B. (2005). VISA is an adapter protein required for virus-triggered IFN-beta signaling. Mol Cell *19*, 727-740.

Xu, W., and Kimelman, D. (2007). Mechanistic insights from structural studies of beta-catenin and its binding partners. J Cell Sci *120*, 3337-3344.

Yamasaki, K., Muto, J., Taylor, K.R., Cogen, A.L., Audish, D., Bertin, J., Grant, E.P., Coyle, A.J., Misaghi, A., Hoffman, H.M., *et al.* (2009). NLRP3/cryopyrin is necessary for interleukin-1beta (IL-1beta) release in response to hyaluronan, an endogenous trigger of inflammation in response to injury. J Biol Chem *284*, 12762-12771.

Yoneyama, M., Kikuchi, M., Matsumoto, K., Imaizumi, T., Miyagishi, M., Taira, K., Foy, E., Loo, Y.M., Gale, M., Jr., Akira, S., *et al.* (2005). Shared and unique functions of the DExD/H-box helicases RIG-I, MDA5, and LGP2 in antiviral innate immunity. J Immunol *175*, 2851-2858.

Yoneyama, M., Kikuchi, M., Natsukawa, T., Shinobu, N., Imaizumi, T., Miyagishi, M., Taira, K., Akira, S., and Fujita, T. (2004). The RNA helicase RIG-I has an essential function in double-stranded RNA-induced innate antiviral responses. Nat Immunol *5*, 730-737.

Yu, H., Li, Q., Kolosov, V.P., Perelman, J.M., and Zhou, X. (2011a). Regulation of cigarette smoke-induced mucin expression by neuregulin1beta/ErbB3 signalling in human airway epithelial cells. Basic Clin Pharmacol Toxicol *109*, 63-72.

Yu, H., Li, Q., Kolosov, V.P., Perelman, J.M., and Zhou, X. (2011b). Regulation of cigarette smoke-mediated mucin expression by hypoxia-inducible factor-1alpha via epidermal growth factor receptor-mediated signaling pathways. J Appl Toxicol.

Zhang, Z., Louboutin, J.P., Weiner, D.J., Goldberg, J.B., and Wilson, J.M. (2005). Human airway epithelial cells sense Pseudomonas aeruginosa infection via recognition of flagellin by Toll-like receptor 5. Infect Immun *73*, 7151-7160.

Zheng, S., De, B.P., Choudhary, S., Comhair, S.A., Goggans, T., Slee, R., Williams, B.R., Pilewski, J., Haque, S.J., and Erzurum, S.C. (2003). Impaired innate host defense causes susceptibility to respiratory virus infections in cystic fibrosis. Immunity *18*, 619-630.

Zheng, S., Xu, W., Bose, S., Banerjee, A.K., Haque, S.J., and Erzurum, S.C. (2004). Impaired nitric oxide synthase-2 signaling pathway in cystic fibrosis airway epithelium. Am J Physiol Lung Cell Mol Physiol *287*, L374-381.

Zhu, L., Lee, P.K., Lee, W.M., Zhao, Y., Yu, D., and Chen, Y. (2009). Rhinovirus-induced major airway mucin production involves a novel TLR3-EGFR-dependent pathway. Am J Respir Cell Mol Biol *40*, 610-619.

Zola, T.A., Lysenko, E.S., and Weiser, J.N. (2008). Mucosal clearance of capsule-expressing bacteria requires both TLR and nucleotide-binding oligomerization domain 1 signaling. J Immunol *181*, 7909-7916.

3

The Role of Alpha–1 Antitrypsin in Emphysema

Sam Alam and Ravi Mahadeva
Department of Medicine, Addenbrooke's Hospital, University of Cambridge
Cambridge
United Kingdom

1. Introduction

Alpha-1 antitrypsin (AT) is a member of the serine proteinase inhibitor (SERPIN) superfamily. It is an acute phase protein produced constitutively, primarily by hepatocytes, and is secreted in to the plasma from where it diffuses into the lung. AT is the most abundant proteinase inhibitor within the lung whose main physiological role is to regulate neutrophil elastase (NE) liberated from activated neutrophils (Brantly et al., 1988a; Lomas and Mahadeva, 2002).

The importance of AT in pulmonary biology was demonstrated by the association between severe plasma deficiency and pulmonary emphysema (Laurell and Eriksson., 1963). These findings in conjunction with Gross et al., 1965 formed the basis of the proteinase-antiproteinase hypothesis for the development of emphysema and other lung diseases. It was subsequently identified that the Z variant is the commonest cause of severe AT deficiency. It results in aggregation of the protein in the hepatocyte (with a predisposition to liver disease) resulting in a secretory defect and deficiency. Initially it was presumed that NE and AT were the most important proteinase and anti-proteinase respectively within the lung, but it is now appreciated that several proteinases and inhibitors exist within the lung and other mechanisms are important e.g. apoptosis, ageing, oxidants. Nevertheless, no other PI and proteinase have been so clearly linked with pulmonary emphysema, thus emphasizing the important role of AT in lung biology. Despite this long association, epidemiological studies suggest that AT deficiency is under-recognized or misdiagnosed (Bull World Health Organ, 1997; ATS-ERS statement, 2003).

1.1 Nomenclature and detection of mutants

The AT protein is an extremely polymorphic molecule; there are over 100 variants of AT resulting from mutations in the *SERPINA1* gene. They are named by the letter of the alphabet according to the migration of the glycosylated form of the protein on isoelectric focusing (IEF). The wildtype protein is therefore termed M-AT as it is associated with normal level of serum AT and it has a medium rate of migration on IEF. Variants that migrate faster than M-AT are classified as A to L or slower than M-AT are classified as N to Z (A being the fastest and Z the slowest) (Brantly et al., 1988a; 1991; Cox et al., 1980; Fagerhol and Laurell, 1967). On the basis of their plasma level and function, the majority of individuals are M homozygotes (M1-5 subtypes).

1.2 Genotyping

Currently, diagnosis of AT deficiency is based on the measurement of AT levels in the serum and/or phenotyping by IEF of the serum within a narrow pH range on the polyacrylamide gel. The latter has been standard practice for many years, but is time consuming, difficult to interpret and limited to a few reference laboratories. Genotyping by real-time PCR and Restriction Fragment-Length Polymorphism PCR (RFLP-PCR) are highly effective, relatively inexpensive and reliable, and as a consequence are now commonly performed. Direct sequencing of coding exons of the gene can also be used as an adjunct in selected cases to clarify genotyping (Zorzetto et al., 2008; Miravitlles et al., 2010).

1.3 Alpha-1-antitrypsin gene expression

The AT gene is located on chromosome 14q31-32.1, and is co-dominantly expressed (Schroeder et al., 1985; Bull World Health Organ, 1997; Brantly et al., 1988). The gene is 12 kb in length and contains seven exons (Ia, b c and II–V) and six introns. Exon I contains the 3′ untranslated promoter sequences: Ia and Ib contains the promoter sequence for macrophage-specific, and Ic for hepatocyte-specific transcription, respectively. The coding regions (Exons II-V) are 1434 base-pairs (bp) in length and the reactive centre is within Exon V (Long et al., 1984). Aside from the promoter elements, there are other regulatory sequences including an enhancer element in the 5' and 3' flanking sequences of exonic regions of the AT gene. A polymorphism in the 3′ flanking region is associated with susceptibility to COPD (Kalsheker et al., 1987; Morgan et al., 1992). A map of single nucleotide polymorphisms (SNPs) in the 5' and 3' flanking regions showed that among the 15 SNPs, five SNPs increased the risk of COPD by 6- to 50-fold (Chappell et al., 2006). These polymorphisms within regulatory sequences are associated with normal basal plasma levels, but can result in reduced levels of AT transcription in response to stimulation *in vitro*, which is postulated to relate to the susceptibility to COPD (Henry et al., 2001; Chappell et al., 2006). However, this has not been proven *in vivo* (Mahadeva et al., 1998; de Faria et al., 2005; Courtney et al., 2006, Brennan, 2007).

1.4 Variants associated with alpha-1 antitrypsin deficiency

The commonest cause of severe deficiency in Caucasians is Z-AT (Glu342Lys). Four percent of North Europeans carry this variant, and amongst them 1/2000 are PiZ homozygotes (Fagerhol, 1974). The frequencies of PiZ are 1/2700 in USA and 1/5000 in UK (Cook, 1975; de Serres, 2002; Brantly et al., 1988a). The distribution of the genetic types (PI alleles) of AT has been investigated in many populations. Some variants are only common in specific populations; the Z mutant is rare in Asian and African populations, whereas the S (364 Glu-Val) variant is more frequent in the Mediterranean area. The plasma level of the principal AT phenotypes are MM (20-39 μmol/L), MS (19-35 μmol/L), SS (14-20 μmol/L), MZ (13-23 μmol/L), SZ (9-15 μmol/L), ZZ (2-8 μmol/L). About 20 variants are associated with lower but detectable AT in plasma (Table 1). The dysfunctional Pittsburgh (M358R) variant converts AT from an elastase inhibitor to a thrombin inhibitor due to mutation in the active site. The Null (QO) variants occur as a result of insertion or deletion of nucleotides. They are associated with only trace amounts (less than 1%) of AT in plasma and associated with increased risk for emphysema (Bull Health World Organ, 1997; ATS-ERS, 2003).

	Variants	Mutations	Mechanism of deficiency	Clinical disease	References
Severe					
	Z	(E342K)	polymerization in liver cells; reduced inhibitory activity; deficiency	Emphysema Liver disease	Oakeshott et al., 1985; Carell, 1990; Ogushi et al., 1987
	Siiyama	(F53S)	polymerization in liver cells and plasma; deficiency	Emphysema Liver disease	Seyama et al., 1991
	Mmalton	(52Phe deleted)	polymerization in liver cells; deficiency	Emphysema Liver disease	Cox and Billingsley, 1989;Roberts et al., 1984
	Mheerlen	(P369L)	intracellular degradation; deficiency	Emphysema	Kramps et al., 1981
	Mprocida	(L41P)	decreased inhibitory activity; deficiency	Emphysema	Takahashi et al., 1988; Holmes et al., 1990 (a)
	P	(D256V)	intracellular degradation; deficiency	Emphysema	Holmes et al., 1990 (b)
	Pittsburgh	(M358R)	altered substrate specificity	Serous bleeding	Owen et al., 1983
Mild					
	S	(E264V)	incorrect splicing of mRNA; abnormal intracellular degradation; polymerization in liver cells		Elliott et al., 1996a; Schindler, 1984; Engh et al., 1989
	I	(R39C)	polymerization; slightly decreased inhibitory activity; mild deficiency	Emphysema	Mahadeva et al., 1999; Graham et al., 1989; Baur and Bencze, 1987
	$M_{mineral\ Springs}$	(G67E)	aberrant posttranslational biosynthesis; loss of conserved Gly; disturbed packing; degraded in liver cells; decreased inhibitory activity; deficiency	Emphysema	Curiel et al., 1990
	F	(R223C)	polymerization; decreased inhibitory activity		Okayama et al., 1991; Hayes et al., 1992

Table 1. Alpha-1-antitrypsin variants associated with plasma deficiency

1.5 Molecular structure of α_1-antitrypsin

AT consists of three β-sheets, eight α-helices, and a reactive centre loop (RCL), which contains the residues that directly interact with the proteinase substrate (Fig. 1). β-Sheet A is composed of five strands spreading along the long axis of the protein: the first strand has 5-6 residues and the other strands have 12-15 residues. In the native conformation, the 17 amino acid RCL locates at an external position in relation to the body of the molecule between the C-terminus of β-sheet A3 and the N-terminus of β-sheet C1. The N-terminal side of the reactive loop including M358 (P1) is directly related to the recognition and binding of the substrate (Fig. 1) (Song et al., 1995; Silverman et al., 2001; Elliott et al., 1996a; Ryu et al., 1996; Kim et al., 2001)

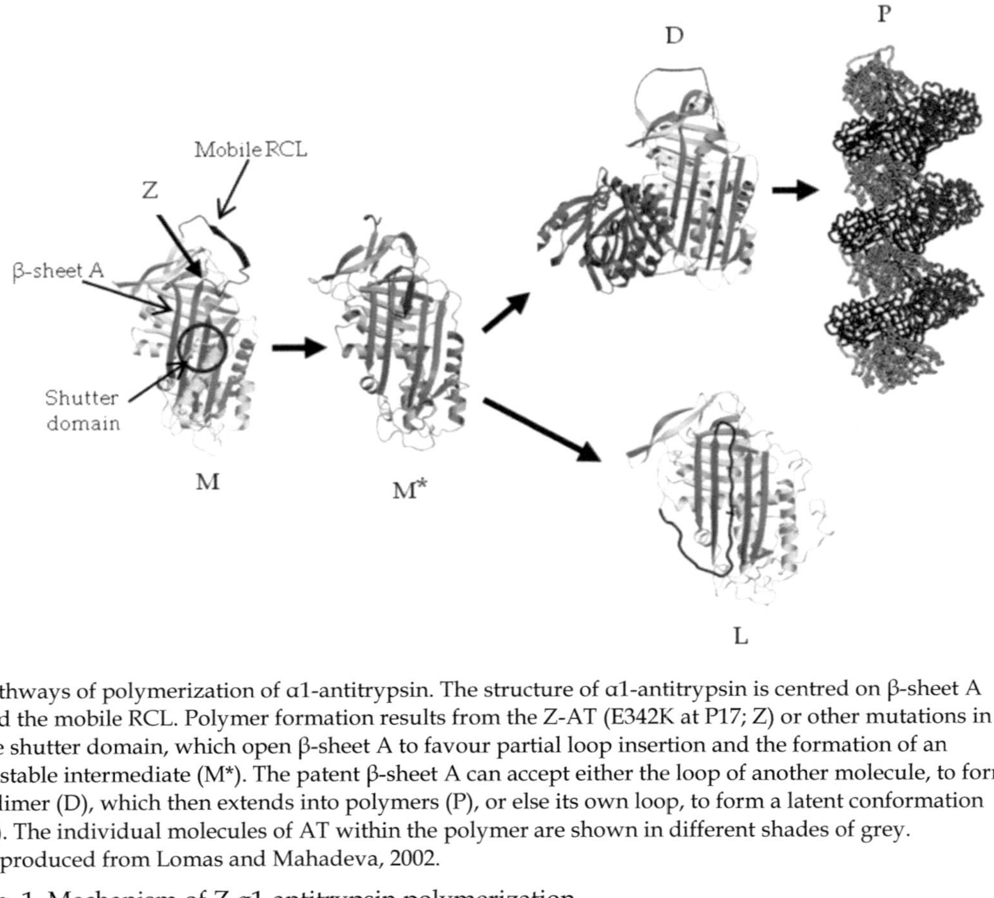

Pathways of polymerization of α1-antitrypsin. The structure of α1-antitrypsin is centred on β-sheet A and the mobile RCL. Polymer formation results from the Z-AT (E342K at P17; Z) or other mutations in the shutter domain, which open β-sheet A to favour partial loop insertion and the formation of an unstable intermediate (M*). The patent β-sheet A can accept either the loop of another molecule, to form a dimer (D), which then extends into polymers (P), or else its own loop, to form a latent conformation (L). The individual molecules of AT within the polymer are shown in different shades of grey. Reproduced from Lomas and Mahadeva, 2002.

Fig. 1. Mechanism of Z α1-antitrypsin polymerization

1.6 Physiology and function of α_1-antitrypsin

AT is a 394 amino acid (52 KDa) glycoprotein produced primarily by hepatocytes. Other cells produce the protein to a lesser extent in peripheral blood monocytes, alveolar macrophages and bronchial epithelial cells and gastrointestinal mucosa. (Brantly et al.,

1988a; Cichy et al., 1997). Daily production of AT is 34 mg/kg. The large amount of AT in the circulation and lung is primarily present to control the activity of elastase in the lung. NE is the main substrate for AT, accordingly it inhibits 90% of the NE in circulation and interstitium of lung. AT also inhibits the serine proteinases cathepsin G and proteinase 3.

1.7 Other biological effects of alpha-antitrypsin

In addition to acting as an antiproteinase, AT plays important role in modulating inflammation. It may inhibit immune responses, and fibroblast-proliferation and fibroblast procollagen production thereby contributing to repair and matrix production (Dabbagh et al., 2001), and have antibacterial activities (Hadzic et al., 2006), and also blocks the cytotoxic and stimulatory activity of defensins (Hiemstra et al., 1998). AT also has direct and indirect anti-apoptotic properties by inhibiting caspase-3 or NE mediated apoptosis, respectively (Petrache et al., 2006). AT is also involved in calcium-induced activation mechanisms; AT inactivates calpain I (μ-calpain), induces a rapid cell polarization and random migration of neutrophils The role of AT in neutrophil regulation was further supported by its ability to transiently increase calcium from intracellular stores, which is linked to neutrophil polarization. AT modulated increase in intracellular lipids, activation of the Rho GTPases, Rac1 and Cdc42, and extracellular signal-regulated kinase (ERK1/2) all these kinases are indeed found to be activated or phosphoryated in polarized neutrophils with significant mobility (Al-Omari et al., 2011). Furthermore, a recent study demonstrated that AT can control immune complex–mediated neutrophil chemotaxis by inhibiting ADAM-17 (TACE) activity and preventing the release of glycosylphosphatidylinositol-linked (GPI-linked) membrane protein, FcγRIIIb, from the cell (Bergin et al., 2010). The same study also demonstrated *in vivo*, that AT is a potent inhibitor of neutrophil chemotaxis in Z-AT individuals compared with M-AT individuals correlating with increased chemotactic responses of both CXCR1 and immune complex receptor (FcγRIIIb) (Bergin et al., 2010).

1.8 Mechanism of proteinase inhibition

The process of inhibition is initiated by the specific binding of the proteinase to the RCL of AT to form a non-covalent Michaelis complex and is one of "suicide substrate inhibition" (Gettins, 2002). The inhibitory mechanism of AT relies upon cleavage of the methionine-serine P1-P1′ by NE (1:1 AT-elastase complex). The protease is then swung 70 Å (1 Å = 0.1 nm) from the upper pole to the lower pole of the protein in association with the insertion of the reactive loop as an extra strand into β-sheet A. The complex inactivates the protease by distortion of the catalytic triad at the active site (Huntington et al., 2000; Wilczynska et al., 1997; Stratikos and Gettins, 1997). The stable complex is subsequently recognized and cleared by the liver. The complexes are short lived (a few hours) in the circulation compared with the native AT (5-6 days), and the low-density lipoprotein receptor related protein (LRP) on liver cells appears to be the principal receptor for clearance of the AT-proteinase complexes (Kounnas et al., 1996).

1.9 Mutations and their effect on conformation of AT

Molecular mobility and the P1 methionine is essential for elastase inhibitory behaviour, but is also its Achilles heel making the molecule vulnerable to the effects of critically situated point mutations and oxidation (Stein and Carrell, 1995). AT molecules can undergo conformational transitions, which not only inactivate is antiproteinase function, but also confers it with other biological properties.

2 Conformations and their effect on structure and function of α_1-antirypsin

2.1 Conformations of α_1-antirypsin

In vivo AT can exist in different conformational forms; native, oxidized, polymerized, oxidized-polymers, RCL cleaved and latent, and the AT-elastase complex. The conformational changes can be the result of inflammation, such as the cleavage by non-target proteinases and oxidation by reactive oxygen species (ROS). Mutaations e.g Z, S predispose it to polymerization. Whilst these conformations result in a loss of proteinase inhibitory activity, they can have biological effects such as inflammatory cell activation and chemotaxis, cytokine release or apoptosis (Janciauskiene, 2001).

2.2 Oxidized AT

Oxidation of AT is a sulphoxide modification of the methionine residues of AT (Johnson and Travis, 1979; Beatty et al., 1980; Taggart et al., 2000). Methionine can be attacked by various oxidants, such as peroxide, hydroxyl radicals, hypochloride, chloramines and peroxynitrite (Vogt, 1995; Rahman and MacNee, 1996), which are mainly produced by activated inflammatory cells. Oxidized AT (Ox-AT) *in vivo* has been confirmed by the finding that the inactive AT purified from the inflammatory synovial fluid contains methionine sulphoxide residues, and that 41% of total AT in the fluid is inactive, oxidized and/or cleaved (Zhang et al., 1993). Smoking is a major external source of oxidants (Rahman and MacNee, 1996; Church and Pryor, 1985; Schaberg et al., 1992). In smoking-related emphysema, 5-10% of total AT is in the oxidized state (Wong and Travis, 1980). Oxidation of the P1 methionine (M358) significantly reduces the activity of AT against NE to 1/2000 of the normal (Johnson and Travis, 1979). Recent data demonstrates that oxidation of Z-AT promotes polymerization of Z-AT thus increasing the risk of emphysema of Z-AT deficient patients (Alam et al., 2011). Ox-AT has also been shown to stimulate release of MCP-1 and IL-8 from lung epithelial cells (Li et al., 2009) and stimulate monocyte activation, inducing an elevation in MCP-1, IL-6, TNF-α expression and NADPH oxidase activity (Moraga and Janciauskiene., 2004)

2.3 Polymerized form

The Z-variant accumulates in the hepatocyte involving a process of loop-sheet polymerization whereby the RCL of one molecule inserts into β-sheet A of a second and so on to form chains of Z-AT polymers (Lomas et al., 1992; Mahadeva et al., 1999). M-AT has not been found to polymerize *in vivo* (Mahadeva et al., 2005). Polymerization can occur in other variants of AT, such as Siiyama, Mmalton, I, and S (Mahadeva et al., 1999; Janciauskiene et al., 2004; Elliott et al., 199b). I α_1-antitrypsin and S-AT polymerize slower than Z-AT but faster than M-AT, and hence are associated with less severe plasma deficiency (Dafforn et al.,1999).

The occurrence of Z-AT polymerization *in vivo* has been confirmed by the finding of AT polymers in lungs (Elliot et al., 1998b; Mulgrew et al., 2004). Polymers of Z-AT are found in emphysematous alveolar walls (Mahadeva et al., 2005). Polymers of Z-AT are chemotactic for neutrophils (Parmar et al., 2002; Mulgrew et al., 2004). Polymers of Z-AT are also ineffective anti-inflammatory molecules or inhibitors of NE, (Alam et al., 2011; Bergin et al., 2010; Al-Omari et al., 2011). Recent findings show that ER accumulation of Z-AT polymers is associated with up-regulation of PKR-like ER kinase (PERK), regulator of G-protein signaling (RGS) 16, and calnexin, and NF-κB activation and secretion of inflammatory mediators; IL-6 and IL-8 in keeping with activation of the ER overload response (EOR) linked to excess inflammatory activity of the Z-AT cell (Alam et al., Unpublished observation).

3. Mechanisms of disease and pathology

3.1 Alpha-1-antitrypsin associated diseases

The normal plasma concentration of AT is about 30 μM, providing 24 μM in lung interstitium, which is thought to be critical in inhibiting elastase. It has been calculated that a concentration of 11 μM of plasma AT is the threshold for providing sufficient AT in the lung (Wewers et al., 1987; Stockely, 2003). Hence, although some phenotypes of AT are associated with abnormally low concentrations of AT in the plasma; PiMS: 80% of normal, PiSS: 60%; PiMZ: 57.5%, only PiSZ, 40%, and PiZ:10-15% and Null variants have been linked to the development of lung disease (Brantly et al., 1988a;b). AT deficiency appears to be under-diagnosed in some populations (Bull World Health Organ, 1997; de Serres, 2003) with only a small proportion of those predicted according to allele frequencies to have AT deficiency to have been identified: 4.5% in UK, 6% in Sweden, and 5% in USA (Tobin et al., 1983; Larsson, 1978; Silverman et al., 1989).

3.2 Z α_1-antitrypsin associated lung disease

Cigarette smoking is the most important independent risk factor for the development of emphysema in the Western world. A landmark study (Fletcher et al., 1977) showed that 15 to 25% of smokers with normal AT develop clinically significant COPD, and that the rate of FEV1 (forced expiratory volume in 1 second) decline was around 50 ml/year in smokers compared with 25 ml/year in non-smokers. Among the AT-deficient population, the decline of FEV1 is 70 ml/year in current smokers compared with 41 ml/year in ex-smokers (Piitulainen and Eriksson, 1999). Smokers with severe deficiency of AT develop symptoms of emphysema 10-15 years earlier than those non-smoking individuals and have a higher mortality (Buist et al., 1983; Janus et al., 1985).

Severe AT deficiency usually due to Z-AT accounts for about 2% of cases of emphysema (Morse, 1978), and has also been linked to asthma and bronchiectasis (Parr et al., 2007; Eden et al., 1997; King et al., 1996; Bleumink and Klokke, 1985). Individuals, who have never smoked, rarely develop symptoms before the age of 50. Twenty-40% of patients have chronic bronchitis and bronchiectasis, and about half have exacerbations (Needham and Stockley, 2004). Most PiZ non-index cases have normal or slightly abnormal lung function in the absence of symptoms (Tobin et al., 1983). The development of lung disease is intimately related to cigarette smoking. However, the severity of lung disease can show some variability: lung function is well maintained in some AT-deficient smokers, while can be impaired in non-smokers (Brantly et al., 1988b; Janus et al., 1985). It is also postulated that host factors, such as individual bronchodilator reversibility, baseline lung function, sex, age, and other unidentified genetic factors as well as other environmental factor such as dust-exposure and recurrent respiratory infections may influence the clinical phenotype (Needham and Stockley, 2004). A recent familial study estimated heritability for FEV_1/forced vital capacity (FVC) in 378 ZZ homozygotes from 167 families identified cigarette smoking as the genetic modifier in the pathogenesis and severity of COPD (DeMeo et al., 2009).

3.3 MZ α_1-antitrypsin associated lung disease

The serum levels of AT in MZ heterozygotes is lower than in MM homozygotes (Section 1.4), but whether MZ individuals have an increased risk of COPD remains controversial. Increased COPD risk in this group may have public health implications because there are about 117 million of MZ and MS phenotypes worldwide (de Serres 2002; Brantly et al., 1991). Many studies have addressed the risk of lung function reduction and increased risk of COPD in MZ heterozygotes, but the results have not been consistent. A meta-analysis demonstrated increased risk of COPD in MZ compared to MM, but there was no difference in mean FEV_1 between MZ and MM individuals when combining the results from population-based studies (Hersh et al., 2004), which is in agreement with a cohort of MZ heterozygotes analyzed from the Danish Alpha-1-Antitrypsin Deficiency Registry (Seersholm et al., 2000) and a longitudinal study of the general population in Arizona (Silva et al., 2003). Many of the previous studies have been limited by small sample sizes, varying phenotype definitions, or failure to adjust for smoking. However, recent studies investigated two large, well characterized populations of current and ex-smokers, a case-control study and a multicenter family-based study using quantitative CT scan measurements of emphysema and airway disease, established an association of reduced FEV_1/FVC in MZ compared to MM (Sandhaus et al., 2008; Sørheim et al., 2010). This suggests that at least some MZ heterozygotes are more susceptible to the development of COPD. Interestingly, MZ with a low smoking history (<20 pack-year) had more severe emphysema on chest CT scan. It remains to be established whether all MZ individuals have an increased risk or whether a subset is more susceptible because of other genetic or environmental factors.

3.4 Mechanism of Z α_1-antitrypsin-related emphysema

The majority of emphysema occurs in cigarette smokers who have normal AT concentrations and smoking can injure the lungs by many mechanisms, such as, A. increasing the oxidant burden (Alam et al., 2011; Church and Pryor, 1985; Carp and Janoff, 1978); B. direct stimulation of neutrophils and macrophages to produce proteinases (Bracke et al., 2005; Hautamaki et al., 1997); C. inactivation of AT and other proteinase inhibitors by oxidation (Alam et al., 2011; Wong and Travis, 1980); D. interfering the repairing process by repeated damage (Janoff et al., 1983). These mechanisms can all occur in Z-AT individuals. However, there are some noteable differences in emphysema due to Z-AT compared to those with normal AT. Firstly, the emphysema has a predilection (although not exclusively) at least initially to affect the lower lobes in Z-AT emphysema compared with the upper lobes in M-AT emphysema. Secondly, the emphysema in Z-AT individuals tends to have more polymorpholeucocytes compared with M-AT emphysema (Morrison et al., 1987).

The main mechanism contributing to the development of emphysema in individuals with Z-AT is the imbalance of AT-elastase, in favour of elastase caused by severe AT deficiency. It is now well established that the conformational changes originating from this mutation predispose Z-AT molecules to irreversible polymerization, with consequent accumulation within the ER of hepatocytes (Lomas et al., 1992; Mahadeva et al., 2002). As a consequence, only approximately 15% of the molecules produced reach the circulation. In addition, in the presence of cigarette smoking a major portion of these secreted proteins has been shown to be either oxidized monomeric AT or in its polymeric form (Alam et al., 2011), which are inactive as proteinase inhibitors. Z-AT also has a reduced activity against elastase (Oakeshhott et al., 1985; Lomas et al., 2003). The inactivation of AT as in M-AT related emphysema can also occur by cleavage by non-target proteinases. The end result of these processes is a further reduction in the quantity of functional AT.

Polymeric conformation of Z-AT has also been found in Z-AT emphysematous lungs in association with neutrophils (Mahadeva et al., 2005). Polymers of Z-AT are also thought to contribute the inflammation and lung damage in emphysema. Polymers of Z-AT are thought to be produced locally within the lung, however, a recent study reported finding of polymers of Z-AT not only in the lung, but also in the serum of transgenic mice expressing human Z-AT that had been exposed to cigarette smoke (Alam et al., 2011) (Section 3.4). Formation of Z-AT polymers may be accelerated by local inflammation e.g. bacterial infection. The polymers are themselves chemotactic for human neutrophils *in vitro* and *in vivo* and are co-localized with neutrophils in the alveoli of individuals with Z-AT-related emphysema (Elliott et al., 1998a; Parmar et al., 2002; Mulgrew et al., 2004). The transition of native Z-AT to polymers inactivates its anti-proteinase and anti-inflammatory function, and also converts it to a pro-inflammatory stimulus and may explain the excess numbers of neutrophils in bronchoalveolar lavage fluid (BALF) and lung tissue from Z-AT homozygotes (Morrison et al., 1987; Mahadeva et al., 2005) and in transgenic Z-AT mice (Alam et al., 2011). The presence of polymers may also contribute to the progression of PiZ lung disease after smoking cessation.

3.5 Cigarette smoking and emphysema

Z-AT related emphysema is potentiated by cigarette smoking, characteristically occurring in the third to fourth decade compared with fifth to sixth decade in non-smokers (Luisetti and Seersholme, 2004; Evald et al., 1990). The mechanism of accelerated decline in smokers with Z-AT is in part due to the independent effects of cigarette smoke, but also due to oxidation of Z-AT which promotes polymerization (production of oxidized polymers) of Z-AT (Fig. 2) (Alam et al., 2011). Polymers are inactive as an anti-elastase, and are not only unable to perform their normal anti-inflammatory role, but are also chemotactic for neutrophils (Alam et al., 2011; Mulgrew et al., 2004; Morrison et al., 1987; Parmar et al., 2002; Bergin et al., 2010; Al-Omari et al., 2011). The acceleration of COPD by cigarette smoke in Z-AT individuals exemplifies the critical importance of gene-environmental interactions to the development of COPD. This provides a molecular explanation for the striking association of premature emphysema in ZZ homozygotes who smoke.

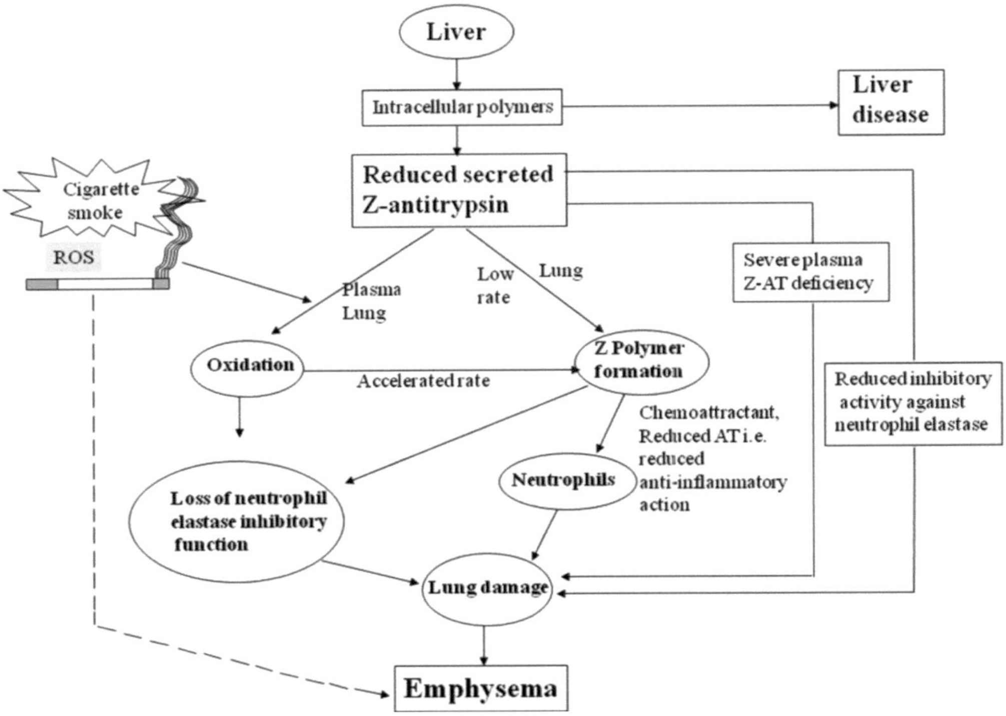

Proposed model for the pathogenesis of emphysema in patients with Z-AT deficiency. Cigarette smoke induces oxidation of Z-AT, which accelerates Z-AT polymerization. Plasma deficiency and reduced inhibitory activity of Z-AT would be exacerbated by the oxidation and polymerization of AT within the lungs, thereby further reducing the antiproteinase screen. Conversion from a monomer to a polymer results in a loss of anti-inflammatory effect. Z-AT polymers also act as a pro-inflammatory stimulus to attract and activate neutrophils, resulting in further increase in neutrophils and liberation of NE thereby imbalance of AT-elastase in the favour of NE leading to tissue damage and subsequently causing emphysema. Adapted from Alam et al., 2011.

Fig. 2. Schematic diagram depicting the role of conformations of α1-antitrypsin and the interaction with cigarette smoke in the development of emphysema.

4. Prognosis and review of current treatments

4.1 Treatment of Z α_1-antitrypsin-associated lung disease

The major goals in the management of patients with Z-AT related emphysema are to prevent lung disease, and to reduce progression of the disease. Smoking cessation and standard management for COPD with normal AT levels is of crucial importance once the diagnosis has been made. Repeated respiratory infections can lead to permanent lung injury in patients with Z-AT deficiency. Thus, reducing exacerbation rate is also essential.

Purified plasma AT (half-life of 4.5 day) and recombinant AT (half-life of a few hours) are both commercially available. Currently four different preparations of purified plasma AT are available worldwide; Prolastin®, Zemaira™, Aralast™ and Trypsone® and have been approved for use by the regulatory agencies in several countries (Table 2). The former three preparations are available in the United States at an estimated cost of $60,000 to $150,000 per year (Gildea et al., 2003). There is no definitive evidence to suggest superiority (specific functional inhibitor activity) of any one of the formulation comparing them to Prolastin. Prolastin was the first approved human purified plasma AT, which is usually administrated intravenously at 60 mg/kg weekly. This dose increased the serum AT level and remained above the putative protective threshold level of 11μM/L after 3 weeks of infusion. However only 2% of the infused purified plasma AT drug reaches to the lung and therefore administration *via* aerosol has also been assessed (Wencker et al., 1998; Hubbard et al., 1989; Smith et al., 1989). Some positive effects of augmentation therapy have been observed in those with moderately impaired lung function (FEV_1 30-65%) (Alpha-1-antitrypsin-Deficiency-Study-Group, 1998; Abusriwil and Stockley, 2006), and some studies have also demonstrated that the treatment reduces airway LTB4, which plays important role in exacerbations (Stockley et al., 2002). However, the therapeutic effect of augmentation therapy is debated due to the lack of a randomized controlled clinical trial (Burrows, 1983; Wewers and Gadek, 1987). There are however problems with conducting such studies: in particular the large numbers of patients with this rare disease required for placebo-controlled and randomized clinical trials; the length of follow-up required to assess efficacy and the limited supply and cost of the treatment (Abusriwil and Stockley, 2006).

Drug	Manufacturer	Method of preparation (viral inactivation)	Minimum specific functional inhibitor activity per mg total protein	Countries approved for use
Prolastin®	Talecris Biotherapeutics, Research Traingle Park, NC	Pasteurization	≥ 0.35 mg	Argentina, Austria, Bahamas, Barbados, Belgium, Bermuda, Canada, Denmark, Finland, Germany, Greece, Guam, Ireland, Italy, Netherlands, Norway, Oman, Poland, Portugal, Puerto Rico, Qatar, Spain, Sweden, Switzerland, US
Zemaira™	CSL Behring, King of Prussia, PA	Pasteurization	≥ 0.7 mg	US
Aralast™ (which was initially called Respitin)	Baxter, Deerfield, IL	Solvent detergent and nanofiltration	≥ 0.55 mg	US
Trypsone®	Grifols, SA.	Solvent detergent and nanofiltration	≥ 0.7 mg	Argentina, Brazil, Chile, Mexico, Spain,

Table 2. Preparations of purified human plasma antitrypsin are available world wide Modrykamien and Stoller, 2009; Stockley et al., 2010; Louie et al., 2005; Barker et al., 1997.

A recent study analyzed results from two randomized, double-blind, placebo-controlled trials to date; a 2-center Danish-Dutch study (n = 54) and the 3-center EXAcerbations and CT scan as Lung Endpoints (EXACTLE) study (n = 65) (Stockley et al., 2010). The study investigated the efficacy of IV AT augmentation therapy on emphysema progression using CT densitometry over an average mean follow-up of about 2.5 years. The study confirmed that IV augmentation therapy significantly reduces the decline in lung density. Decline from baseline to last CT scan was -4.082 g/L versus -6.379 g/L for placebo, with the treatment difference of 2.297 (95% CI, 0.669 to 3.926; p=0.006), the corresponding annual declines were -1.73 and -2.74 g/L/yr, respectively) and may therefore reduce the future risk of mortality in patients with AT deficiency related emphysema, in favour of IV AT augmentation therapy.

There is no evidence that IV augmentation therapy with purified plasma AT preparations is effective in MZ genotypes. MZ patients are at risk for accelerated airflow obstruction/lung disease as mentioned above and that augmentation therapy in MZ patients can be associated with side effects (Stoller et al., 2003/2009). The Medical and Scientific Advisory Committee of the Alpha-1 Foundation (Sandhaus et al., 2008) concluded that augmentation therapy for MZ phenotypes should be avoided.

4.2 Alpha-1 antitrypsin deficiency and Lung volume reduction surgery

Recently lung volume reduction surgery (LVRS) has been proposed as a treatment for severe emphysema. Over the years studies reported both in favour and against LVRS in AT deficient patients (Dauriat et al., 2006; Tutic et al., 2004). Because LVRS offers only short-term benefits for most AT deficient patients LVRS should not be recommended in these patients pending additional studies (ATS–ERS, 2003). This data is further supported by landmark studies from the National Emphysema Treatment Trial (NETT) (Fishman et al 2003; Stoller et al 2007) that included 1218 randomized subjects and 10 who were randomized had severe Z-AT deficiency and underwent LVRS. Deficient individuals had a shorter duration in FEV_1 rise, smaller increase in exercise capacity at 6 months, and higher mortality (20% vs. 0% compared with medical treatment) after 2 years. Although these conclusions are inherently limited by the small number of patients analyzed, LVRS cannot clearly be recommended for this population based on the above data (Stoller et al 2007). In addition, most patients with Z-AT deficiency have lower lobe predominant emphysema, which showed the least surgical benefit in NETT (leading to worse outcomes in good exercise capacity patients) (Stoller et al 2007). Although LVRS has small functional gains and a shorter-lasting effect in AT deficient patients than in patients with normal AT emphysema, it could potentially serve as a bridging procedure that postpones the need for lung transplantation (Dauriat et al., 2006; Tutic et al., 2004). Emerging techniques for bronchoscopic lung volume reduction are covered in another chapter.

4.3 Alpha-1 antitrypsin deficiency and Lung transplantation

End stage pulmonary emphysema is the most common indication for lung transplantation worldwide. Lung transplantation is considered in patients with declining lung function or symptomatic patients with a poor quality of life after receiving all conservative treatment options including smoking cessation and rehabilitation programmes. A functional improvement and better quality of life are clear benefits deriving from lung transplantation, while a survival advantage has not yet been proven (Marulli and Rea, 2008). Studies have shown advantage of single versus double lung transplantation for COPD or AT deficiency. However, a common cause of death PiZ post transplantation was due to pulmonary infection and bronchiolitis obliterans syndrome (BOS), and sepsis in the presence of excess NE (Meyer et al., 2001; Tanash et al., 2011; de Perrot et al., 2004). A recent study analyzed a total of 83 PiZZ patients with severe emphysema who underwent lung transplantation between 1990 and June 2010 compared to 70 age, gender, smoking history and lung function matched controls (Tanash et al., 2011). Of 83 transplanted patients, 62 (75%) underwent single-lung transplantation. During follow-up, 37 (45%) deaths occurred in transplanted patients and 45 (64%) in the non transplanted patients. In the transplanted patients, the estimated median survival time was 11 years (95% confidence interval [CI] 9 to 14 years), compared with 8 years (95% CI 4 to 6 years) for the non transplanted patients ($p = 0.006$) (Tanash et al., 2011). Constant annual death rates due to BOS and other complications result in a 50% 5-year survival (Patterson and Cooper, 1995). In addition, Mal and colleagues (Mal et al., 2004) have shown an association between cigarette smoking induced NE activity and recurrence of pulmonary emphysema in the transplanted lung of a 49 year old PiZ patient 11 years after receiving single lung transplant. Therefore, lung transplantation should only be offered to selected candidates.

4.4 Treatment of Z α1-antitrypsin-associated liver disease

A major distinction between pathogenesis of lung and liver disease in Z-AT deficiency is loss of function and gain of function, respectively. In liver disease it relates to the intracellular accumulation of misfolded and unsecreted AT from hepatocytes rather than unopposed elastolysis in the lung due to lack of AT. Therefore, augmentation therapy does not confer protect against and not indicated for liver disease relating to severe AT deficiency. Other strategies have been assessed for treatment of Z-AT related liver disease including targeting a lateral hydrophobic cavity to prevent polymerization, and enhancing clearance of Z-AT aggregates by drugs promoting autophagy (Zhou et al., 2004; Burrows et al., 2000; Mallya et al., 2007; Hedvegi et al., 2010; Devlin et al., 2001; Kaushal et al., 2010). These methods reduce intracellular aggregation of Z-AT but do not increase the secretion Z-AT. Use of short synthetic peptides targeting β-sheet A may show therapeutic potential for Z-AT related liver and lung disease (Figure 3) (Chang et al., 2006; 2009; Alam et al., Unpublished observation).

5. Novel treatments in development

5.1 Gene therapy

Future therapies for α_1-antitrypsin deficiency include gene therapy. Supplementing AT by gene delivery is an alternative way to increase the local AT in lung. Preclinical studies have shown that the Adeno-associated viral vector is capable in increasing the AT concentration to over 11μM in the lung. The safety and efficiency of this approach is under evaluation (Flotte, 2002; Flotte et al., 2004; Stecenko and Brigham, 2003; Flotte and Mueller, 2011).

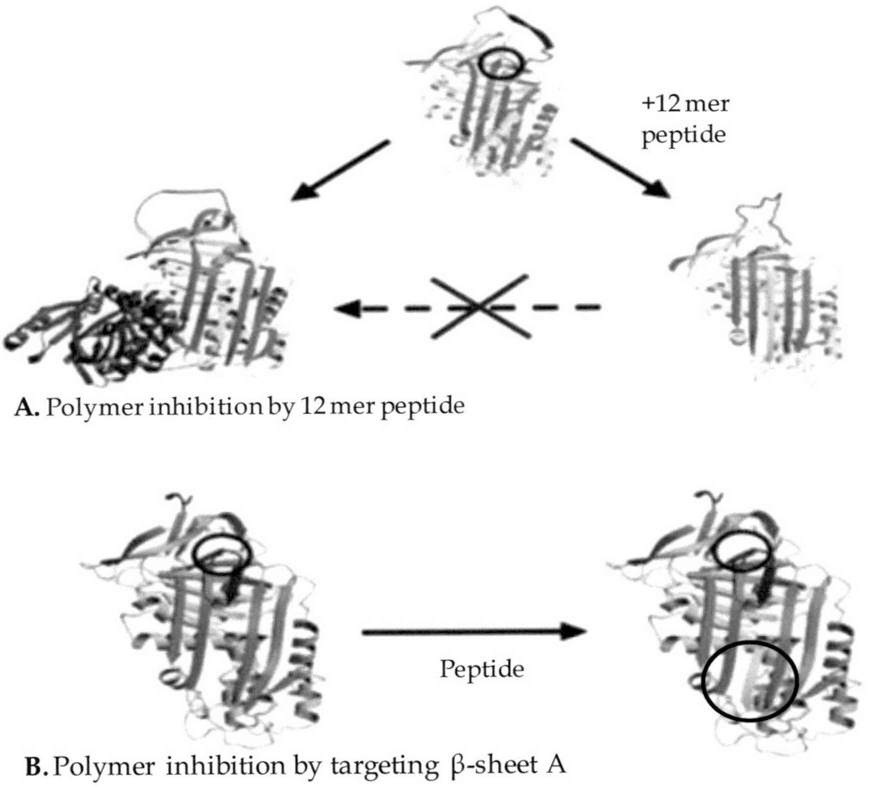

A. Z mutation (E342K) perturbs the structure of AT to allow opening of β-sheet A, which then accepts the RCL of another molecule to form a dimer (*left*) that can extend to form chains of polymers as depicted in Fig. 1. 12-mer peptide can anneal to β-sheet A thereby preventing polymer formation (*right*). B. Z mutation allows partial insertion of the RCL. This opens the lower part of β-sheet A thereby favouring polymerization (*left*). Understanding the configuration of the reactive loop and interacting with β-sheet A prompted the hypothesis that a 6-mer with homology to P_{7-2} of the RCL would specifically bind to Z-AT and so prevent polymerization and explained why the 12-mer peptide preferentially bound to M-AT (*right*). Reproduced and adapted from Lomas and Mahadeva, 2002; Mahadeva et al., 2002; Chang et al., 2009.

Fig. 3. Representation Z α1-antitrypsin polymerization and the design of a selective inhibitor.

6. Summary

Alpha-1-antitrypsin is the most important proteinase inhibitor in maintaining the proteinase/antiproteinase balance within the lung. The recognition of the association between plasma deficiency of α1-antitrypsin and emphysema over 40 years ago has led to the proteinase-antiproteinase hypothesis of lung disease which remains central to understanding lung biology. In the last 20 years there has been significant progress in our understanding of α1-antitrypsin. Alpha-1 antitrypsin may modulate other biological processes such as apoptosis and inflammatory cell recruitment. Z α1-antitrypsin polymerizes within the liver and this accounts for its severe plasma deficiency, and α1-antitrypsin polymers may have a role in the progression of emphysema, but this requires further investigation. Recent and ongoing studies should clarify the role of augmentation therapy and lung volume reduction in subgroups of PiZZ homozygotes, and the understanding of polymer formation has raised the exciting prospect of developing new therapeutic strategies for the liver and lung disease associated with Z α1-antitrypsin.

7. References

Abusriwil, H. & Stockley, R. A. (2006) *Cur Opin Pul Med* 12(2), 125-131

Alam, S., Li, Z., Janciauskiene, S. & Mahadeva, R. (2011) *Am J Respir Cell Mol Biol* 45(2):261-269.

Alam, S., Wang, J., Janciauskiene, S. & Mahadeva R, (2011) (Unpublished observation).

Al-Omari, M., Korenbaum, E., Ballmaier, M., Lehmann, U., Jonigk, D., Manstein, D. J., Welte, T., Mahadeva, R. & Janciauskiene, S. (2011) *Mol Med.* [Epub ahead of print]

Alpha-1-antitrypsin-Deficiency-Registry-Study-Group. (1998) *Am J Respir Crit Care Med* 158(1)

ATS-ERS; American Thoracic Society/European Respiratory Society statement (2003) *Am J Respir Crit Care Med* 168(7):818-900.

Barker, A.F., Iwata-Morgan, I., Oveson, L. & Roussel R. (1997) *Chest* 112(4):872-4.

Baur, X. & Bencze, K. (1987) *Respir* 51(3), 188-195

Beatty, K., Bieth, J. & Travis J. (1980) *J Biol Chem* 255: 3931–3934.

Bergin, D. A., Reeves, E. P., Meleady, P., Henry, M., McElvaney, O. J., Carroll, T. P., Condron, C., Chotirmall, S. H., Clynes, M., O'Neill, S. J. & McElvaney, N. G. (2010) *J Clin Invest* 120(12):4236-5420.

Bleumink, E. & Klokke, A. H. (1985) *Arch Dermatol Res* 1985;277(4):328-9.

Bracke, K., Cataldo, D., Maes, T., Gueders, M., Noel, A., Foidart, J. M., Brusselle, G. & Pauwels, R. A. (2005) *Int Arch Allerg and Imm* 138(2), 169-179

Brantly, M., Nukiwa, T. & Crystal, R. G. (1988a) *Am J Med* 84(6A), 13-31

Brantly, M. L., Paul, L. D., Miller, B. H., Falk, R. T., Wu, M. & Crystal, R. G. (1988b) *Am Rev Respir Dis* 138(2), 327-336

Brantly, M. L., Wittes, J. T., Vogelmeier, C. F., Hubbard, R. C., Fells, G. A. & Crystal, R. G. (1991) *Chest* 100(3):703-708.

Brennan, S. (2007) *Eur Respir J* 29(2), 229-230

Bull World Health Organ (1997) 75(5):397–415.

Buist, A. S., Burrows, B., Eriksson, S., Mittman, C., & Wu, M. (1983) *Am Rev Resp Dis* 127(2), S43-45

Burrows, B. (1983) *Am Rev Respir Dis* 127(2), S42-43

Burrows, J. A., Willis, L. K. & Perlmutter, D. H. (2000) *PNAS USA* 97(4), 1796-1801

Carell, R. W. (1990) *Lung* 168 Suppl, 530-534

Carp, H. & Janoff, A. (1978) *Am Rev Resp Dis* 118(3), 617-621

Chang, Y. P., Mahadeva, R., Chang, W. S., Shukla, A., Dafforn, T. R., & Chu, Y. H. (2006)*Am J Respir Cell Mol Biol* 35(5), 540-548

Chang, Y. P., Mahadeva, R., Chang, W. S., Lin, S. C. & Chu, Y. H. (2009) *J Cell Mol Med* 13(8B):2304-2316.

Chappell, S., Daly, L., Morgan, K., Guetta Baranes, T., Roca, J., Rabinovich, R., Millar, A., Donnelly, S. C., Keatings, V., MacNee, W., Stolk, J., Hiemstra, P., Miniati, M., Monti, S., O'Connor, C. M. & Kalsheker, N. (2006) *Hum Mut* 27(1), 103-109

Church, D. F. & Pryor, W. A. (1985) *Environ Health Perspect* 64, 111-126

Cichy, J., Potempa, J. & Travis, J. (1997) *J Biol Chem* 272(13):8250-8255.

Cook, P. J. (1975) *Ann Hum Genet* 38(3):275-87.

Courtney, J. M., Plant, B. J., Morgan, K., Rendall, J., Gallagher, C., Ennis, M., Kalsheker, N., Elborn, S. & O'Connor, C.M. (2006) *Ped Pul* 41(6), 584-591

Cox, D. W. & Billingsley, G. D. (1989) *Am J Hum Genet* 44(6), 844-854

Cox, D. W., Johnson, A. M. & Fagerhol, M.K. (1980) *Hum Genet* 53:429–433.

Curiel, D. T., Vogelmeier, C., Hubbard, R. C., Stier, L. E. & Crystal, R. G. (1990) *Mole Cell Biol* 10(1), 47-56

Dabbagh, K., Laurent, G. J., Shock, A., Leoni, P., Papakrivopoulou, J., and Chambers, R. C. (2001) *J Cell Physiol* 186(1), 73-81

Dafforn, T. R., Mahadeva, R., Elliott, P. R., Sivasothy, P., and Lomas, D. A. (1999) *J Biol Chem* 274(14), 9548-9555

Dauriat, G., Mal, H., Jebrak, G., Brugière, O., Castier, Y., Camuset, J., Marceau, A., Taillé, C., Lesèche, G. & Fournier, M. (2006) *Int J Chron Obstruct Pulmon Dis* 1(2):201-6.

de Faria, E. J., de Faria, I. C., Alvarez, A. E., Ribeiro, J. D., Ribeiro, A. F. & Bertuzzo, C. S. (2005) *J Pediat (Rio J)* 81(6), 485-490

DeMeo, D. L., Campbell, E. J., Brantly, M. L., Barker, A. F., Eden, E,. McElvaney, N. G., Rennard, S. I., Stocks, J. M., Stoller, J. K., Strange, C., Turino, G., Sandhaus, R. A. & Silverman, E. K. *Hum Hered.* 2009;67(1):38-45.

de Perrot, M., Chaparro, C., McRae, K., Waddell, T. K., Hadjiliadis, D., Singer, L. G., Pierre, A. F., Hutcheon, M. & Keshavjee, S. (2004) *J Thorac Cardiovasc Surg* 127(5):1493-501.

de Serres, F. J. (2002) *Chest* 122(5):1818-1829.

de Serres, F. J. (2003) *Environ Health Perspect* 111(16), 1851-1854

Devlin, G. L., Parfrey, H., Tew, D. J., Lomas, D.A. & Bottomley, S.P. (2001) *Am J Respir Cell Mol Biol* 24:727–732.

Elliott, P. R., Abrahams, J. P. & Lomas, D. A. (1998a) *J Mol Biol* 275(3), 419-425

Elliott, P. R., Bilton, D. & Lomas, D. A. (1998b) *Am J Resp Cell Mol Biol* 18(5), 670-674

Elliott, P. R., Lomas, D. A., Carrell, R. W., and Abrahams, J. P. (1996a) *Nat Struct Biol* 3(8), 676-681

Elliott PR, Stein PE, Bilton D, Carrell RW, Lomas DA. (1996b) *Nat Struct Biol* 3(11):910-911.

Engh, R., Lobermann, H., Schneider, M., Wiegand, G., Huber, R. & Laurell, C. B. (1989) *Prot Eng* 2(6), 407-415

Evald, T., Dirksen, A., Keittelmann, S., Viskum, K. & Kok-Jensen, A. (1990) *Lung* 168 Suppl, 579-585.

Fagerhol, M. K. (1974) *Birth defects original article series* 10(4), 208-211

Fagerhol, M. K. & Laurell, C. B. (1967) *Clin Chim Acta* 16(2), 199-203

Fishman, A., Martinez, F., Naunheim, K., Piantadosi, S., Wise, R., Ries, A., Weinmann, G. & Wood, D. E; National Emphysema Treatment Trial Research Group. (2003) *N Engl J Med* 348(21):2059-73.

Fletcher, A. P., Alkjaersig, N. K., O'Brien, J. R., & Tulevski, V. (1977) *J Lab Clin Med* 89(6), 1349-1364

Flotte, T. R. (2002) *Chest* 121(3 Suppl), 98S-102S

Flotte, T. R., Brantly, M. L., Spencer, L. T., Byrne, B. J., Spencer, C. T., Baker, D. J. & Humphries, M. (2004) *Hum Gen Therp* 15(1), 93-128
Flotte, T. R. & Mueller, C. (2011) *Hum Mol Genet* 20(R1):R87-92.
Gettins, P. G. (2002) *Chem Rev* 102(12):4751-4804.
Gildea, T. R., Shermock, K. M., Singer, M. E. & Stoller, J. K. (2003) *Am J Respir Crit Care Med* 167:1387–1392
Graham, A., Kalsheker, N. A., Newton, C. R., Bamforth, F. J., Powell, S. J. & Markham, A. F. (1989) *Hum Genet* 84(1), 55-58
Hautamaki, R. D., Kobayashi, D. K., Senior, R. M. & Shapiro, S. D. (1997) *Sci (New York, N.Y* 277(5334), 2002-2004
Hayes, K., Graham, A., & Kalsheker, N. (1992) *Biochem Soc Trans* 20(2), 182S
Hadzic, R., Nita, I., Tassidis, H., Riesbeck, K., Wingren, A. G. & Janciauskiene, S. (2006) *Immunol Lett* 102:141-147.
Henry, M. T., Cave, S., Rendall, J., O'Connor, C. M., Morgan, K., FitzGerald, M. X. & Kalsheker, N. (2001) *Eur J Hum Genet* 9(4), 273-278
Hersh, C. P., Dahl, M., Ly, N. P., Berkey, C. S,. Nordestgaard, B. G. & Silverman, E. K. (2004) *Thorax* 59(10): 843-849.
Hidvegi, T., Schmidt, B. Z., Hale, P. & Perlmutter, D. H. (2005) *J Biol Chem* 280(47), 39002-39015
Hidvegi, T., Ewing, M., Hale, P., Dippold, C., Beckett, C., Kemp, C., Maurice, N., Mukherjee, A., Goldbach, C., Watkins, S., Michalopoulos, G., Perlmutter, D. H. (2010) *Sci* 329(5988):229-232.
Hiemstra, P., Wetering, S. van, & Stolk, J. (1998) *Eur Respir J* 12
Hodges, J. R., Millward-Sadler, G. H., Barbatis, C. & Wright, R. (1981) *N Engl J Med* 304(10), 557-560
Holmes, M. D., Brantly, M. L. & Crystal, R. G. (1990a) *Am Rev Respir Dis* 142(5), 1185-1192
Holmes, M. D., Brantly, M. L., Fells, G. A. & Crystal, R. G. (1990b) *BBRC* 170(3), 1013-1020
Hubbard, R. C., McElvaney, N. G., Sellers, S. E., Healy, J. T., Czerski, D. B. & Crystal, R. G. (1989) *J Clin Invest* 84(4), 1349-1354
Huntington, J. A., Read, R. J. & Carrell, R. W. (2000) *Nature* 407(6806), 923-926
Janciauskiene, S. (2001) *Biochim Biophys Acta* 1535(3):221-35.
Janciauskiene, S., Eriksson, S., Callea, F., Mallya, M., Zhou, A., Seyama, K., Hata, S. & Lomas D. A. (2004) *Hepatol* 40(5):1203-10.
Janoff, A., Carp, H., Laurent, P. & Raju, L. (1983) *Am Rev Respir Dis* 127(2), S31-38
Janus, E. D., Phillips, N. T. & Carrell, R. W. (1985) *Lancet* 1(8421), 152-154
Johnson, D. & Travis, J. (1979) *J Biol Chem* 254(10):4022-6.
Kalsheker, N. A., Hodgson, I. J., Watkins, G. L., White, J. P., Morrison, H. M. & Stockley, R. A. (1987) *Br Med J (Clin Res Ed)* 294(6586), 1511-1514
Kim, S., Woo, J., Seo, E. J., Yu, M. & Ryu, S. (2001) *J Mol Biol* 306(1), 109-119
King, M. A., Stone, J. A., Diaz, P. T., Mueller, C. F., Becker, W. J. & Gadek JE. (1996) *Radiol* 199(1):137-41.
Kounnas, M. Z., Church, F. C., Argraves, W. S. & Strickland, D. K. (1996) *J Biol Chem* 271(11), 6523-6529
Kaushal, S., Annamali, M., Blomenkamp, K., Rudnick, D., Halloran, D., Brunt, E.M., & Teckman, J. H. (2010) *Exp Biol Med* 235(6):700-709.
Kramps, J. A., Brouwers, J. W., Maesen, F. & Dijkman, J. H. (1981) *Hum Genet* 59(2), 104-107

Larsson, C. (1978) *Acta Med Scand* 204(5), 345-351

Laurell, C. B. & Eriksson, S. (1963) *Scand J Clin Invest* 15;132-140.

Li, Z., Alam, S., Wang, J., Sandstrom, C. S., Janciauskiene, S. & Mahadeva, R. (2009) *Am J Physiol Lung Cell Mol Physiol* 297:L388-400.

Lomas, D. A., Evans, D. L., Stone, S. R., Chang, W. S. & Carrell, R. W. (1993) *Biochem* 19;32(2):500-8.

Lomas, D. A. & Mahadeva, R. (2002) *J Clin Invest* 110(11), 1585-1590

Lomas, D. A., Evans, D. L., Finch, J. T. & Carrell, R. W. (1992) *Nature* 357(6379), 605-607

Long, G. L., Chandra, T., Woo, S. L., Davie, E. W., & Kurachi, K. (1984) *Biochem* 23(21), 4828-48370-280

Louie, S. G., Sclar, D. A. & Gill, M. A. (2005) *Ann Pharmacother* 39(11):1861-1869.

Lu, Q., Harrington, E. O. & Rounds, S. (2005) *Keio J Med* 54(4), 184-189

Luisetti, M. & Seersholm, N. (2004) *Thorax* 59(2):164-9.

Mahadeva, R. & Lomas, D. A. (1998) *Thorax* 53(6), 501-505

Mahadeva, R., Atkinson, C., Li, Z., Stewart, S., Janciauskiene, S., Kelley, D. G., Parmar, J., Pitman, R., Shapiro, S. D. & Lomas, D. A. (2005) *Am J Path* 166(2), 377-386

Mahadeva, R., Westerbeek, R. C., Perry, D. J., Lovegrove, J. U., Whitehouse, D. B., Carroll, N. R., Ross-Russell, R. I., Webb, A. K., Bilton, D. & Lomas, D. A. (1998) *Eur Respir J* 11(4):873-9

Mahadeva, R., Chang, W. S., Dafforn, T. R., Oakley, D. J., Foreman, R. C., Calvin, J., Wight, D. G., & Lomas, D. A. (1999) *J Clin Invest* 103(7), 999-1006

Mahadeva, R., Dafforn, T. R., Carrell, R. W. & Lomas, D. A. (2002) *J Biol Chem* 277(9), 6771-6774

Mal, H., Guignabert, C., Thabut, G., d'Ortho, M. P., Brugière, O., Dauriat, G., Marrash-Chahla, R., Rangheard, A. S., Lesèche, G. & Fournier, M. (2004) *Am J Respir Crit Care Med* 170(7):811-814

Mallya, M., Phillips, R. L., Saldanha, S. A., Gooptu, B., Brown, S. C., Termine, D. J., Shirvani, A. M., Wu, Y., Sifers, R. N., Abagyan, R. & Lomas, D. A. (2007) *J Med Chem* 50(22):5357-5363.

Meyer, K. C., Nunley, D. R., Dauber, J. H., Iacono, A. T., Keenan, R. J., Cornwell, R. D. & Love, R. B. (2001) *Am J Respir Crit Care Med* 164(1):97-102.

Miravitlles, M., Herr, C., Ferrarotti, I., Jardi, R., Rodriguez-Frias, F., Luisetti, M. & Bals, R. (2010) *Eur Respir J* 35(5):960-8

Modrykamien, A. & Stoller, J. K. (2009) *Pharmacother* 10(16):2653-2661.

Moraga, F. & Janciauskiene, S. (2000) *J Biol Chem* 275(11), 7693-7700

Morgan, K., Scobie, G. & Kalsheker, N. (1992) *Eur J Clin Invest* 22(2), 134-137

Morrison, H. M., Kramps, J. A., Burnett, D. & Stockley, R. A. (1987) *Clin Sci* (Lond). 72:373-381

Morse, J. O. (1978) *N Engl J Med* 299(20), 1099-1105

Mulgrew, A. T., Taggart, C. C., Lawless, M. W., Greene, C. M., Brantly, M. L., O'Neill, S. J., & McElvaney, N. G. (2004) *Chest* 125(5), 1952-1957

Needham, M., & Stockley, R. A. (2004) *Thorax* 59(5), 441-445

Oakeshott, J. G., Muir, A., Clark, P., Martin, N. G., Wilson, S. R. & Whitfield, J. B. (1985) *Ann Hum Biol* 12(2), 149-160

Ogushi, F., Fells, G. A., Hubbard, R. C., Straus, S. D. & Crystal, R. G. (1987) *J Clin Invest* 80(5), 1366-1374

Okayama, H., Brantly, M., Holmes, M. & Crystal, R. G. (1991) *Am J Hum Genet* 48(6), 1154-1158

Owen, C. A., Campbell, M. A., Sannes, P. L., Boukedes, S. S. & Campbell, E. J. (1995) *J Cell Biol* 131(3), 775-789

Owen, M. C., Brennan, S. O., Lewis, J. H. & Carrell, R. W. (1983) *N Engl J Med* 309(12), 694-698

Patterson, G. A. & Cooper, J. D. (1995) *Chest Surg Clin N Am* 5(4):851-68.

Parmar, J. S., Mahadeva, R., Reed, B. J., Farahi, N., Cadwallader, K. A., Keogan, M. T., Bilton, D., Chilvers, E. R. & Lomas, D. A. (2002) *Am J Respir Cell Mol Biol* 26(6), 723-730

Parr, D. G., Guest, P. G., Reynolds, J. H., Dowson, L. J. & Stockley, R. A. (2007) *Am J Respir Crit Care Med* 176(12):1215-21.

Petrache, I., Fijalkowska, I., Medler, T. R., Skirball, J., Cruz, P., Zhen, L., Petrache, H. I., Flotte, T. R. & Tuder, R. M. (2006) *Am J Pathol* 169(4), 1155-1166

Piitulainen, E. & Eriksson, S. (1999) *Eur Respir J* 13(2), 247-251

Rahman, I. & MacNee, W. (1996) *Free Rad Biol Med* 21(5), 669-681

Roberts, E. A., Cox, D. W., Medline, A. & Wanless, I. R. (1984) *Am J Clin Pathol* 82(4), 424-427

Ryu, S. E., Choi, H. J., Kwon, K. S., Lee, K. N. & Yu, M. H. (1996) *Struct* 4(10), 1181-1192

Sandhaus, R. A., Turino, G., Stocks, J., Strange, C., Trapnell, B. C., Silverman, E. K., Everett, S. E. & Stoller, JK; *Chest* 134(4):831-834.

Schindler, D. (1984) In Human Genetic Disorders: 16t' Miami Winter Symposium. In: S. Ahmad, S. B., J. Schulz, W. Scott, and J. Whelan (ed). *Advances in Gene Technology*, Cambridge University Press, Cambridge

Schroeder, W. T., Miller, M. F., Woo, S. L. & Saunders, G. F. (1985) *Am J Hum Genet* 37(5), 868-872

Seersholm, N., Wilcke, J. T., Kok-Jensen, A. & Dirksen, A. (2000) *Am J Respir Crit Care Med* 161(1):81-84.

Seyama, K., Nukiwa, T., Takabe, K., Takahashi, H., Miyake, K. & Kira, S. (1991) *J Biol Chem* 266(19), 12627-12632

Silva, G. E., Sherrill, D. L., Guerra, S. & Barbee, R.A. (2003) *Chest* 123(5):1435-1440.

Silverman, E. K., Miletich, J. P., Pierce, J. A., Sherman, L. A., Endicott, S. K., Broze, G. J., Jr., & Campbell, E. J. (1989) *Am Rev Respir Dis* 140(4), 961-966

Silverman, G. A., Bird, P. I., Carrell, R. W., Church, F. C., Coughlin, P. B., Gettins, P. G., Irving, J. A., Lomas, D. A., Luke, C. J., Moyer, R. W., Pemberton, P. A., Remold-O'Donnell, E., Salvesen, G. S., Travis, J. & Whisstock, J. C. (2001) *J Biol Chem* 276:33293–33296.

Smith, R. M., Traber, L. D., Traber, D. L. & Spragg, R. G. (1989) *J Clinic Invest* 84(4), 1145-1154

Song, H. K., Lee, K. N., Kwon, K. S., Yu, M. H. & Suh, S. W. (1995) *FEBS Lett* 377(2), 150-154

Sørheim, I. C., Bakke, P., Gulsvik, A., Pillai, S. G., Johannessen, A., Gaarder, P. I., Campbell, E. J., Agustí, A., Calverley, P. M., Donner, C. F., Make, B. J., Rennard, S. I., Vestbo, J., Wouters, E. F., Paré, P. D., Levy, R. D., Coxson, H. O., Lomas, D. A., Hersh, C. P. & Silverman, E. K. (2010) *Chest* 138(5):1125-1132.

Stratikos, E. & Gettins, P. G. (1997). *Proc Natl Acad Sci USA* 94: 453-458.

Stein, P. E. & Carrell, R. W. (1995) *Nat Struct Biol* 2(2), 96-113

Stecenko, A. A. & Brigham, K. L. (2003) *Gene Ther* 10(2):95-9.

Stockley, R. A. (2010) *Expert Opin Emerg Drugs* 15(4):685-94.

Stockley, R. (2003) Antiproteinases and antioxidants. In: Gibson GJ, G. D., Costabel U, Sterk, P, and Corrin B. (ed). *Respir Med*, Third Ed., Elsevier Science limited, London

Stockley, R. A., Parr, D. G., Piitulainen, E., Stolk, J., Stoel, B. C. & Dirksen, A. (2010) *Respir Res* 11:136

Stockley, R. A., Bayley, D. L., Unsal, I. & Dowson, L. J. (2002) *Am J Respir Crit Care Med* 165(11), 1494-1498

Stoller, J. K., Fallat, R., Schluchter, M. D., O'Brien, R. G., Connor, J. T., Gross, N., O'Neil, K., Sandhaus, R. & Crystal, R. G. 2003 / *Chest* 2009 136(5 Suppl):e30

Stoller, J. K., Fallat, R., Schluchter, M. D., O'Brien, R. G., Connor, J. T., Gross, N., O'Neil, K., Sandhaus, R. & Crystal, R. G. (2003) *Chest* 123(5):1425-34

Stoller, J. K., Gildea, T. R., Ries, A. L., Meli, Y. M. & Karafa, M. T; National Emphysema Treatment Trial Research Group. (2007) *Ann Thorac Surg* 83(1):241-51.

Sveger, T. (1976) *N Engl J Med* 294(24), 1316-1321

Taggart, C., Cervantes-Laurean, D., Kim, G., McElvaney, N. G., Wehr, N., Moss, J. & Levine, R. L. (2000) *J Biol Chem* 275: 27258-27265.

Takahashi, H. & Crystal, R. G. (1990) *Am J Hum Genet* 47(3), 403-413

Takahashi, H., Nukiwa, T., Satoh, K., Ogushi, F., Brantly, M., Fells, G., Stier, L., Courtney, M. & Crystal, R. G. (1988) *J Biol Chem* 263(30), 15528-15534

Tanash, H. A., Riise, G. C., Hansson, L., Nilsson, P. M. & Piitulainen, E. *J Heart Lung Transplant* 2011 Aug 5. [Epub ahead of print]

Tobin, M. J., Cook, P. J. & Hutchison, D. C. (1983) *Brit J Dis chest* 77(1), 14-27

Tutic, M., Bloch, K. E., Lardinois, D., Brack, T., Russi, E. W. & Weder, W. (2004) *J Thorac Cardiovasc Surg* 128(3):408-13.

Vogt, W. (1995) *Free Rad Biol Med* 18(1), 93-105

Wencker, M., Banik, N., Hotze, L. A., Kropp, J., Biersack, M. J., Ulbich, E. & Konietzko, N. *Am J Respir Crit Care Med* 1998;154:A400.

Wewers, M. D. & Gadek, J. E. (1987) *Ann Intern Med* 107(5), 761-763

Wewers, M. D., Casolaro, M. A. & Crystal, R. G. (1987) *Am Rev Respir Dis* 135(3), 539-543

Wilczynska, M., Fa, M., Karolin, J., Ohlsson, P. I., Johansson, L. B. & Ny, T. (1997) *Nat Struct Biol* 4(5):354-7.

Wong, P. S. & Travis, J. (1980) *BBRC* 96(3), 1449-1454

Zhang, Z., Farrell, A. J., Blake, D. R., Chidwick, K. & Winyard, P. G. (1993) *FEBS Lett* 321(2-3), 274-278

Zhou, A., Stein, P. E., Huntington, J. A., Sivasothy, P., Lomas, D. A. & Carrell, R. W. (2004) *J Mol Biol* 342(3), 931-941

Zorzetto, M., Russi, E., Senn, O., Imboden, M., Ferrarotti, I., Tinelli, C., Campo, I., Ottaviani, S., Scabini, R., von Eckardstein, A., Berger, W., Brändli, O., Rochat, T., Luisetti, M. & Probst-Hensch, N; SAPALDIA Team. (2008) *Clin Chem* 54(8):1331-1338.

4

The Dichotomy Between Understanding and Treating Emphysema

Frank Guarnieri
Paka Pulmonary Pharmaceuticals, Acton, Department of Physiology and Biophysics, MA, School of Medicine, Virginia Commonwealth University, Richmond, VA, Department of Biomedical Engineering, Boston University, Boston, MA, USA

1. Introduction

The long history of investigations into the causes and potential treatments of emphysema encompasses a vast array of chemical and biological research disciplines. A key finding that played a major role in initiating these inquiries occurred in 1963 when Laurell and Eriksson[1] found that individuals with a genetic deficiency in serum alpha-1-antitrypsin (AAT) were prone to develop pulmonary emphysema[2]. This genetic linkage was given a mechanistic basis when Turino and colleagues in 1969 discovered that patients with reduced inhibition of pancreatic elastase also lacked serum AAT and were prone to develop severe pulmonary emphysema[3]. Subsequent studies in the early 1970s confirmed that excessive elastase activity due to lack of AAT was in fact the genetic mechanism responsible for the onset of emphysema [4-7]. A key environmental connection was made with the discovery that cigarette smoke increased macrophage secretion of elastase[8] in the lungs, oxidized AAT[9], and that the chemical irritants in smoke recruited neutrophils to the lungs via chemotaxis[10-12]. This integrated genetic-environmental understanding firmly established elastase inhibition as a mechanistic target for preventing the alveolar destruction characteristic of emphysema.

The validation of elastase[13, 14] as a protein target for treating emphysema, motivated three different therapeutic approaches, 1) infusing patients with AAT purified from serum[15], 2) development of small molecule inhibitors[13, 16, 17], 3) novel association of small peptides[18] and synthetic inhibitors [19] with albumin microspheres. The first approach is a biological therapeutic, the second approach is a chemical therapeutic, and the third approach is a prescient recognition that *in vivo* efficacy will likely require long lung residence time pharmacodynamics. The Pharmaceutical industry launched several major multi-decade programs to develop orally available small molecule inhibitors, while apparently completely ignoring the concurrent academic medical research beginning to unravel the complex biology of emphysema and its indication that oral delivery of small molecules was unlikely to have any therapeutic benefit. Interestingly, a completely different basic research discipline, X-ray crystallography, had a seminal impact on the class of molecules from which Zeneca derived their clinical candidate. The first structure[20] was solved In 1976 by Alber, Petsko, and Tsernoglou, which showed atomic resolution details of elastase digesting a substrate. Sawyer and colleagues deposited the first high resolution crystal structure of porcine pancreatic elastase[21] into the protein data bank, and in 1982 Hughes and colleagues[22] solved a structure of the enzyme bound to a trifluoroacetyl dipeptide inhibitor (deposited in the PDB in 1986), thus making high resolution structures with and without bound ligand available to the research community. The trifluoroacetyl motif (shown in Figure 1) became a cornerstone of Zeneca's small molecule research program[23-32], which resulted in the clinical candidate ICI 200,880[33]that was halted due to lack of efficacy in Phase II clinical trials.

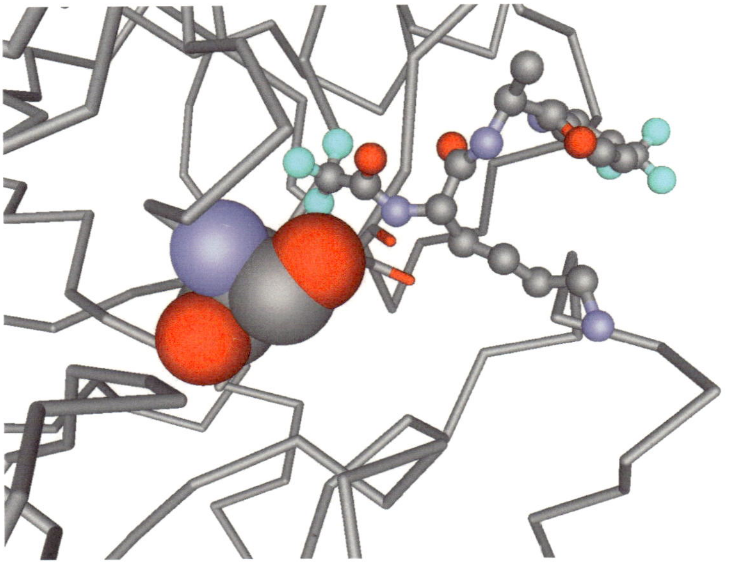

Fig. 1. Co-crystal structure taken from the protein data bank file 2EST. This structure shows the catalytic serine (shown in space fill) performing a nucleophilic attack on the carbon of the ketone attached to a trifluoromethyl group - the fluorines are shown in light blue. The highly electronegative fluorine atoms significantly enhance the electropositive nature of this carbon and hence trifluoromethyl-ketone molecules have a high affinity for elastase.

Even as the first therapeutics were being developed, a report on neutrophil lung recruitment via elastin peptide chemotaxis [34] gave the first indications of the complexity and immunological involvement [35] in the development of pulmonary diseases. Elastase digests elastin resulting in peptide fragments that elicit circulating neutrophils to enter the lungs. These neutrophils secrete fresh elastase causing new lung damage, new elastin peptide fragments and recruitment of new neutrophils again secreting fresh elastase into the lungs in a destructive feedback loop. These studies already presented evidence that inhibiting elastase in the short term would be insufficient to treat emphysema. Compounding the complexity, early elastase inhibitors administered intraperitoneally that showed promise in stemming emphysema, cleared rapidly [36] *in vivo* with concomitant renal nephropathy [17]. The complex interplay between lung injury and immune response that begins with a single intratrachael instillation of elastase motivated many detailed studies aimed at elucidating the basic biology of emphysema progression. Early key findings on the long term effects on lung tissue of only one exposure to elastase includes, 1) ultrastructural changes occurring 16 days later [37], 2) dose related changes in pulmonary function after 4 weeks [38], 3) 14 day lung residence time of the enzyme complexed with alpha-macroglobulin [39], 4) resistance to AAT inactivation in the presence of activated neutrophils [40], 5) uptake by alveolar macrophages with subsequent re-release of elastase [41]. Additionally, activated neutrophils can secrete elastase for over 12 days [42].

2. Lessons from the Stone lab

While the complex biology of emphysema most likely precludes treatment using a simple small molecule elastase inhibitor strategy, important physiological parameters essential for developing an effective therapeutic modality were reported by Stone and Lucey between 1988 and 1991. These investigators showed that, 1) one intratracheal dose of elastase causes maximum damage after 4 weeks [43], 2) a potent elastase inhibitor given intratracheally in 170-fold molar excess has a lung half-life of 4 minutes (Figure 2) and actually results in worse emphysema relative to animals given saline with no elastase [44], 3) covalently linking an active small molecule to a polymer of hydroxyethyl-aspartamide (stationary phase for hydrophilic column chromatography) results in a lung half-life of 441 minutes and amelioration of elastase induced emphysema [45]. This collection of results indicates that long lung residence time is an essential component of any meaningful emphysema treatment and that elastase must be down-regulated continuously for at least 4 weeks.

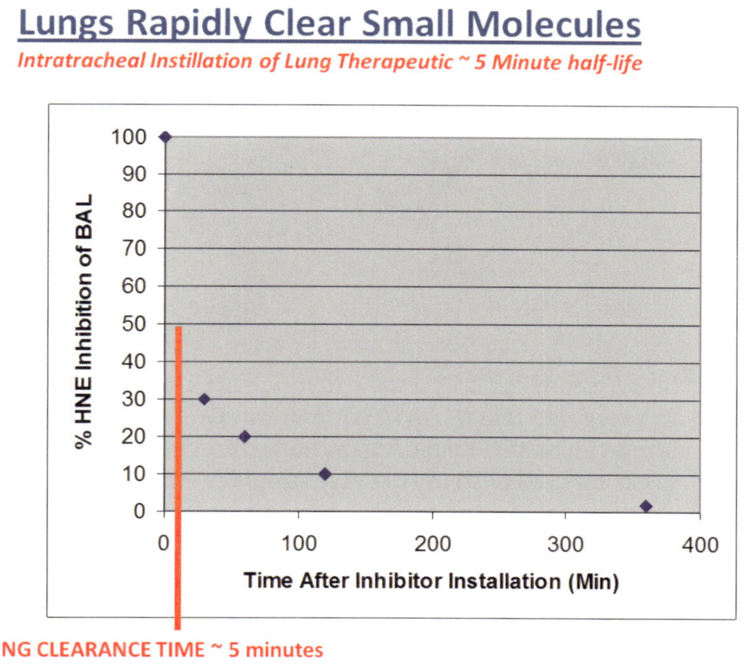

Fig. 2. This is a recreation of the data from Phil Stone's lab showing that small molecule elastase inhibitors have a lung half-life of 4-5 minutes. It is important to understand that these experiments were conducted by intratracheally instilling the small molecule elastase inhibitor and thus 100% of the dose was initially deposited into the lungs. Small molecules administered orally will result in only a tiny fraction of the dose ever actually entering the lungs.

3. Combining inhibitors with surfactant replacement therapy

Even though Zeneca's clinical candidate ICI 200,880 was halted in Phase II clinical trials for lack of human efficacy, the molecule possessed two essential features of a drug, 1) high affinity anti-elastase activity, and 2) it was deemed safe to give to humans as evidenced by passing Phase I clinical trials. When the small molecule chemistry work of Zeneca is combined with the *in vivo* biology work of Phil Stone, the logical conclusion is that an efficacious *in vivo* emphysema treatment requires that ICI 200,880 somehow be recast so that it spreads across the vast surface area of the lungs and resists being expelled into systemic circulation. If such a recasting could be achieved, the long lung residence time could result in an immune response, thus ultimately negating the treatment. So the next logical step places the strong constraint that any adjuvant molecule used to do the recasting must naturally reside in the lungs. A natural lung molecule that has the intrinsic properties of spreading across the vast surface area of the lungs is a defining property of the lung surfactants.

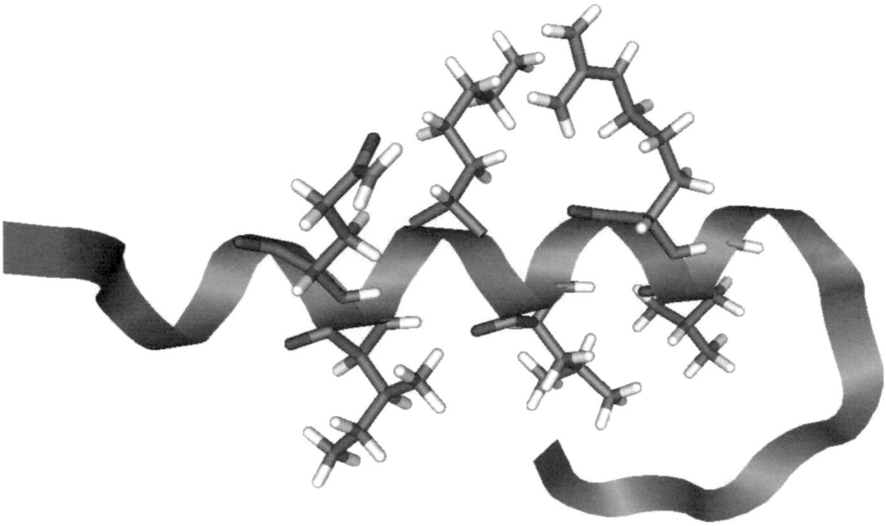

Fig. 3. NMR structure of residues 1-25 from the N-terminal of surfactant peptide B taken from the protein data bank file 1DFW. An important feature of this peptide is its amphiphilic structure as illustrated by having one face composed of hydrophobic residues and the opposite face composed of charged and hydrophilic amino acids.

Human lung surfactant is a complex mixture of lipids and peptides that was extensively studied in the 1980s when it was realized that delivering surfactant harvested from animals to the lungs of severely pre-term infants is a life-saving [46-52] procedure. Early biophysical studies of lung surfactant indicated that it was ~90% lipids and ~10% protein by weight [53]. Detailed analysis showed that the protein component was actually made up of 4 different molecules, 2 larger hydrophilic proteins and 2 smaller hydrophobic proteins [54, 55]. Remarkably, when 1% or 0.1% by weight of the smallest of these proteins isolated from lavage fluid was added to synthetic phospholipids, both mixtures essentially eliminated dynamic surface tension in biophysical experiments [56, 57], a result that the investigators admitted was truly startling. The protein with such astounding surface active properties is a 79 residue peptide now called surfactant protein B. What is even more amazing is that subsequent biophysical studies demonstrated that the first 25 amino acids possesses essentially identical surface active properties[58, 59] to the whole protein (Figure 3). Further confirmation of the importance of the first domain of surfactant protein B comes from Discovery Labs with their Phase III clinical studies that one dose of (Lys-Leu-Leu-Leu)$_4$ [60] a mimetic of SP-B 1-25 added to cow lavage dramatically reduces mortality in severely preterm infants [61].

4. Conclusion

The long, involved, complicated history of emphysema integrates genetics, protein and small molecule therapies, medicinal chemistry, crystallography, biophysics, and several other research disciplines. Interestingly, all of this complexity can lead to a rather simple conclusion - that covalently linking Zeneca's clinical candidate to the first 25 residues of surfactant peptide B (Figure 4) would be an effective long acting anti-emphysema treatment if delivered intratracheally. When these studies were carried out[62], one dose of the SP-B (1-25)-Zeneca peptide-small molecule construct completely protected rodents exposed to near lethal doses of the human neutrophil elastase for 4 weeks (Figures 5&6). Of course it remains to be seen whether or not this simple idea will prove to be efficacious in humans, because recent studies have demonstrated that AAT plays a complex multifactorial role in the recruitment of neutrophils into the lungs. For example, Li[63] and colleagues have demonstrated that oxidized AAT induces lung epithelial cells to release IL-8, resulting in CXCR1 mediated neutrophil chemotaxis into the lungs, while Bergin[64] and coworkers have shown that glycosylated AAT sequesters IL-8 disrupting activation of CXCR1 and neutrophil mobilization. To further complicate matters, calpain[65] induces TNF-alpha mediated neutrophil chemotaxis and AAT binds to and inhibits calpain[66] thus preventing lung neutrophil infiltration by yet another mechanism. Even with all of this complexity and its implications that antioxidant therapy may be beneficial, the long established destructive role of unchecked elastase activity makes this enzyme a central target for inhibiting the progression of the alveolar wall destruction characteristic of emphysema as evidenced by the extensive pharmaceutical development that has gone into this endeavor, which includes small molecules from ONO[67], Merck[68], Zeneca[24], and Glaxo[69] (Figure 7).

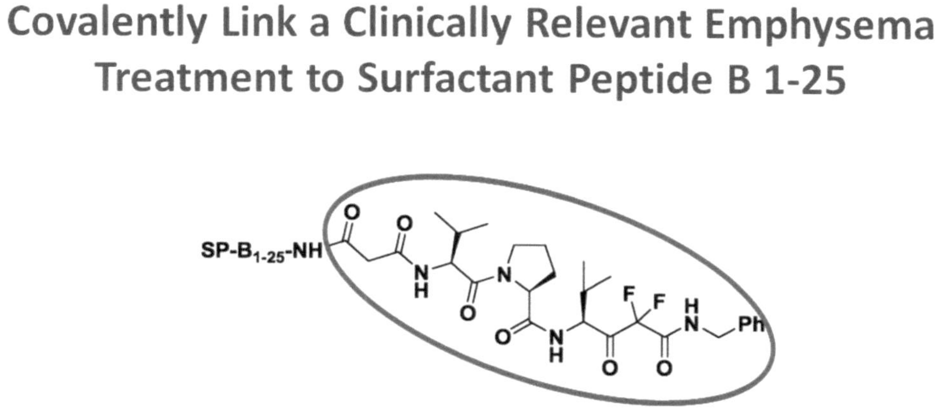

Fig. 4. A small molecule from the Zeneca family of fluoro-peptidomimetics covalently linked to the N-terminal of the first 25 residues of surfactant peptide B.

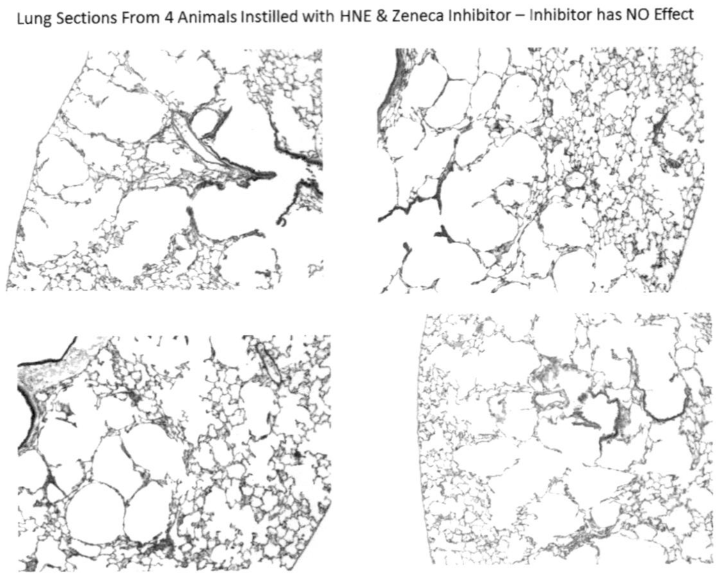

Fig. 5. Emphysema is induced in rodents by intratracheally instilling human neutrophil elastase. When elastase is administered with a potent Zeneca small molecule inhibitor, the rodents develop emphysema after 4 weeks to the same degree as rodents given no inhibitor. The small molecule was in 70-fold molar excess concentration relative to elastase.

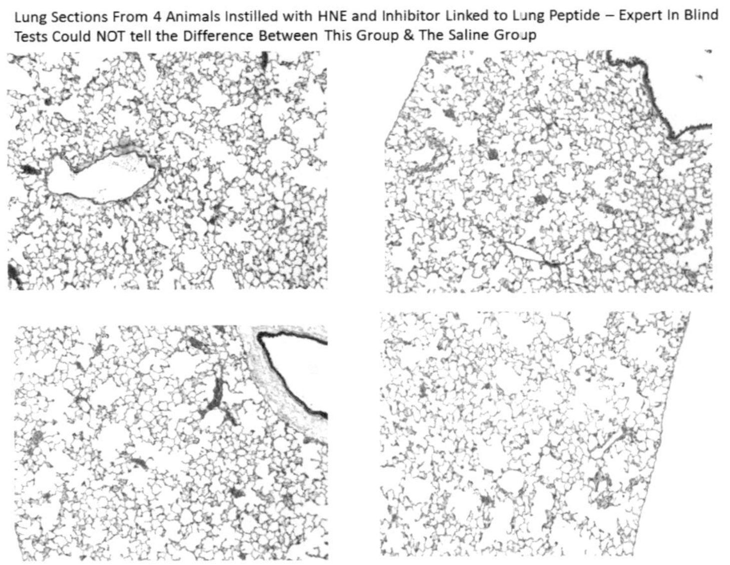

Fig. 6. When this exact same small molecule was covalently linked to the fragment of surfactant peptide B as shown in Figure 4, one dose given in 30 fold molar excess completely protected the animal for 4 weeks. All animals were dosed with a mixture of HNE and either the Zeneca small molecule or the Zeneca small molecule covalently attached to the surfactant peptide and sacrificed after 4 weeks.

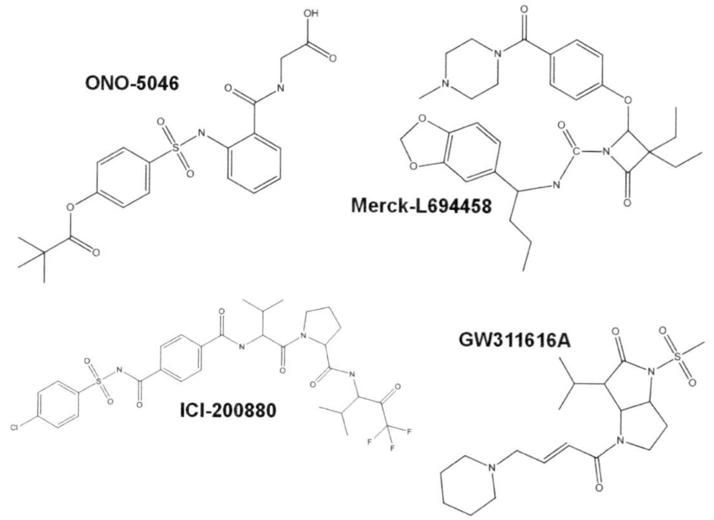

Fig. 7. Small molecule elastase inhibitors from ONO, Merck, Zeneca, and Glaxo.

5. References

[1] Laurell, C.B. and S. Eriksson, *The electrophoretic alpha-iglobulin pattern of serum in alpha-1-antitrypsin deficiency.* Scand. J. Clin. Lab. Invest., 1963. 15: p. 132-140.

[2] Kueppers, F., W.A. Briscoe, and A.G. Bearn, *Hereditary Deficiency of Serum Alpha-L-Antitrypsin.* Science, 1964. 146: p. 1678-9.

[3] Turino, G.M., et al., *Serum elastase inhibitor deficiency and alpha 1-antitrypsin deficiency in patients with obstructive emphysema.* Science, 1969. 165(894): p. 709-11.

[4] Lieberman, J., *Involvement of leukocytic proteases in emphysema and antitrypsin deficiency.* Arch Environ Health, 1973. 27(3): p. 196-200.

[5] Mittman, C., T. Barbela, and J. Lieberman, *Antitrypsin deficiency and abnormal protease inhibitor phenotypes.* Arch Environ Health, 1973. 27(3): p. 201-6.

[6] Pierce, J.A., A.Z. Eisen, and H.K. Dhingra, *Relationship of antitrypsin deficiency to the pathogenesis of emphysema.* Trans Assoc Am Physicians, 1969. 82: p. 87-97.

[7] Talamo, R.C., et al., *Symptomatic pulmonary emphysema in childhood associated with hereditary alpha-1-antitrypsin and elastase inhibitor deficiency.* J Pediatr, 1971. 79(1): p. 20-6.

[8] Harris, J.O., et al., *Comparison of proteolytic enzyme activity in pulmonary alveolar macrophages and blood leukocytes in smokers and nonsmokers.* Am Rev Respir Dis, 1975. 111(5): p. 579-86.

[9] Janoff, A. and H. Carp, *Possible mechanisms of emphysema in smokers: cigarette smoke condensate suppresses protease inhibition in vitro.* Am Rev Respir Dis, 1977. 116(1): p. 65-72.

[10] Gadek, J.E., G.A. Fells, and R.G. Crystal, *Cigarette smoking induces functional antiprotease deficiency in the lower respiratory tract of humans.* Science, 1979. 206(4424): p. 1315-6.

[11] Janoff, A., et al., *Cigarette smoke inhalation decreases alpha 1-antitrypsin activity in rat lung.* Science, 1979. 206(4424): p. 1313-4.

[12] Rodriguez, R.J., et al., *Elastase release from human alveolar macrophages: comparison between smokers and nonsmokers.* Science, 1977. 198(4314): p. 313-4.

[13] Janoff, A. and R. Dearing, *Prevention of elastase-induced experimental emphysema by a synthetic elastase inhibitor administered orally.* Bull Eur Physiopathol Respir, 1980. 16 Suppl: p. 399-405.

[14] Kleinerman, J., et al., *The effect of the specific elastase inhibitor, alanyl alanyl prolyl alanine chloromethylketone, on elastase-induced emphysema.* Am Rev Respir Dis, 1980. 121(2): p. 381-7.

[15] Gadek, J.E., et al., *Replacement therapy of alpha 1-antitrypsin deficiency. Reversal of protease-antiprotease imbalance within the alveolar structures of PiZ subjects.* J Clin Invest, 1981. 68(5): p. 1158-65.

[16] Lange, F., et al., *Comparative effects of reversible and irreversible specific elastase inhibitors on elastase-induced emphysema.* Bull Eur Physiopathol Respir, 1980. 16 Suppl: p. 407-13.

[17] Ranga, V., et al., *Effects of oligopeptide chloromethylketone administered after elastase: renal toxicity and lack of prevention of experimental emphysema.* Am Rev Respir Dis, 1981. 124(5): p. 613-8.

[18] Martodam, R.R., et al., *Albumin microspheres as carrier of an inhibitor of leukocyte elastase: potential therapeutic agent for emphysema.* Proc Natl Acad Sci U S A, 1979. 76(5): p. 2128-32.

[19] Gudapaty, S.R., et al., *The prevention of elastase-induced emphysema in hamsters by the intratracheal administration of a synthetic elastase inhibitor bound to albumin microspheres.* Am Rev Respir Dis, 1985. 132(1): p. 159-63.

[20] Alber, T., G.A. Petsko, and D. Tsernoglou, *Crystal structure of elastase-substrate complex at -- 55 degrees C.* Nature, 1976. 263(5575): p. 297-300.

[21] Sawyer, L., et al., *The atomic structure of crystalline porcine pancreatic elastase at 2.5 A resolution: comparisons with the structure of alpha-chymotrypsin.* J Mol Biol, 1978. 118(2): p. 137-208.

[22] Hughes, D.L., et al., *Crystallographic study of the binding of a trifluoroacetyl dipeptide anilide inhibitor with elastase.* J Mol Biol, 1982. 162(3): p. 645-58.

[23] Veale, C.A., et al., *Orally active trifluoromethyl ketone inhibitors of human leukocyte elastase.* J Med Chem, 1997. 40(20): p. 3173-81.

[24] Edwards, P.D., et al., *Discovery and biological activity of orally active peptidyl trifluoromethyl ketone inhibitors of human neutrophil elastase.* J Med Chem, 1997. 40(12): p. 1876-85.

[25] Edwards, P.D., et al., *Nonpeptidic inhibitors of human neutrophil elastase. 7. Design, synthesis, and in vitro activity of a series of pyridopyrimidine trifluoromethyl ketones.* J Med Chem, 1996. 39(5): p. 1112-24.

[26] Edwards, P.D., et al., *Peptidyl alpha-ketoheterocyclic inhibitors of human neutrophil elastase. 3. In vitro and in vivo potency of a series of peptidyl alpha-ketobenzoxazoles.* J Med Chem, 1995. 38(20): p. 3972-82.

[27] Veale, C.A., et al., *Nonpeptidic inhibitors of human leukocyte elastase. 5. Design, synthesis, and X-ray crystallography of a series of orally active 5-aminopyrimidin-6-one-containing trifluoromethyl ketones.* J Med Chem, 1995. 38(1): p. 98-108.

[28] Veale, C.A., et al., *Non-peptidic inhibitors of human leukocyte elastase. 4. Design, synthesis, and in vitro and in vivo activity of a series of beta-carbolinone-containing trifluoromethyl ketones.* J Med Chem, 1995. 38(1): p. 86-97.

[29] Bernstein, P.R., et al., *Nonpeptidic inhibitors of human leukocyte elastase. 6. Design of a potent, intratracheally active, pyridone-based trifluoromethyl ketone.* J Med Chem, 1995. 38(1): p. 212-5.

[30] Bernstein, P.R., et al., *Nonpeptidic inhibitors of human leukocyte elastase. 3. Design, synthesis, X-ray crystallographic analysis, and structure-activity relationships for a series of orally*

active 3-amino-6-phenylpyridin-2-one trifluoromethyl ketones. J Med Chem, 1994. 37(20): p. 3313-26.

[31] Damewood, J.R., Jr., et al., *Nonpeptidic inhibitors of human leukocyte elastase. 2. Design, synthesis, and in vitro activity of a series of 3-amino-6-arylopyridin-2-one trifluoromethyl ketones.* J Med Chem, 1994. 37(20): p. 3303-12.

[32] Warner, P., et al., *Non-peptidic inhibitors of human leukocyte elastase. 1. The design and synthesis of pyridone-containing inhibitors.* J Med Chem, 1994. 37(19): p. 3090-9.

[33] Edwards, P.D. and P.R. Bernstein, *Synthetic inhibitors of elastase.* Med Res Rev, 1994. 14(2): p. 127-94.

[34] Senior, R.M., G.L. Griffin, and R.P. Mecham, *Chemotactic activity of elastin-derived peptides.* J Clin Invest, 1980. 66(4): p. 859-62.

[35] Hunninghake, G.W. and J.E. Gadek, *Immunological aspects of chronic non-infectious pulmonary diseases of the lower respiratory tract in man.* Clin Immunol Rev, 1981. 1(3): p. 337-74.

[36] Ip, M.P., et al., *The effects of small doses of oligopeptide elastase inhibitors on elastase-induced emphysema in hamsters: a dose-response study.* Am Rev Respir Dis, 1981. 124(6): p. 714-7.

[37] Morris, S.M., et al., *Ultrastructural changes in hamster lung four hours to twenty-four days after exposure to elastase.* Anat Rec, 1981. 201(3): p. 523-35.

[38] Raub, J.A., et al., *Dose response of elastase-induced emphysema in hamsters.* Am Rev Respir Dis, 1982. 125(4): p. 432-5.

[39] Stone, P.J., et al., *Role of alpha-macroglobulin-elastase complexes in the pathogenesis of elastase-induced emphysema in hamsters.* J Clin Invest, 1982. 69(4): p. 920-31.

[40] Zaslow, M.C., et al., *Human neutrophil elastase does not bind to alpha 1-protease inhibitor that has been exposed to activated human neutrophils.* Am Rev Respir Dis, 1983. 128(3): p. 434-9.

[41] McGowan, S.E., et al., *The fate of neutrophil elastase incorporated by human alveolar macrophages.* Am Rev Respir Dis, 1983. 127(4): p. 449-55.

[42] Werb, Z. and S. Gordon, *Elastase secretion by stimulated macrophages. Characterization and regulation.* J Exp Med, 1975. 142(2): p. 361-77.

[43] Lucey, E.C., et al., *An 18-month study of the effects on hamster lungs of intratracheally administered human neutrophil elastase.* Exp Lung Res, 1988. 14(5): p. 671-86.

[44] Stone, P.J., E.C. Lucey, and G.L. Snider, *Induction and exacerbation of emphysema in hamsters with human neutrophil elastase inactivated reversibly by a peptide boronic acid.* Am Rev Respir Dis, 1990. 141(1): p. 47-52.

[45] Lucey, E.C., et al., *A polymer-bound elastase inhibitor is effective in preventing human neutrophil elastase-induced emphysema.* Ann N Y Acad Sci, 1991. 624: p. 341-2.

[46] Halliday, H.L., *Clinical experience with exogenous natural surfactant.* Dev Pharmacol Ther, 1989. 13(2-4): p. 173-81.

[47] Halliday, H.L., et al., *Acute effects of instillation of surfactant in severe respiratory distress syndrome.* Arch Dis Child, 1989. 64(1 Spec No): p. 13-6.

[48] Long, W., et al., *A controlled trial of synthetic surfactant in infants weighing 1250 g or more with respiratory distress syndrome. The American Exosurf Neonatal Study Group I, and the Canadian Exosurf Neonatal Study Group.* N Engl J Med, 1991. 325(24): p. 1696-703.

[49] Robertson, B., *Surfactant replacement in neonatal and adult respiratory distress syndrome.* Eur J Anaesthesiol, 1984. 1(4): p. 335-43.

[50] Robertson, B., *Neonatal respiratory distress syndrome and surfactant therapy; a brief review.* Eur Respir J Suppl, 1989. 3: p. 73s-76s.

[51] Vidyasagar, D., et al., *Surfactant replacement therapy: clinical and experimental studies.* Clin Perinatol, 1987. 14(3): p. 713-36.

[52] Vidyasagar, D. and S. Shimada, *Pulmonary surfactant replacement in respiratory distress syndrome.* Clin Perinatol, 1987. 14(4): p. 991-1015.

[53] Yu, S., et al., *Bovine pulmonary surfactant: chemical composition and physical properties.* Lipids, 1983. 18(8): p. 522-9.

[54] Ross, G.F., et al., *Phospholipid binding and biophysical activity of pulmonary surfactant-associated protein (SAP)-35 and its non-collagenous COOH-terminal domains.* J Biol Chem, 1986. 261(30): p. 14283-91.

[55] Whitsett, J.A., et al., *Hydrophobic surfactant-associated protein in whole lung surfactant and its importance for biophysical activity in lung surfactant extracts used for replacement therapy.* Pediatr Res, 1986. 20(5): p. 460-7.

[56] Notter, R.H. and D.L. Shapiro, *Lung surfactants for replacement therapy: biochemical, biophysical, and clinical aspects.* Clin Perinatol, 1987. 14(3): p. 433-79.

[57] Notter, R.H., et al., *Biophysical activity of synthetic phospholipids combined with purified lung surfactant 6000 dalton apoprotein.* Chem Phys Lipids, 1987. 44(1): p. 1-17.

[58] Gupta, M., et al., *Comparison of functional efficacy of surfactant protein B analogues in lavaged rats.* Eur Respir J, 2000. 16(6): p. 1129-33.

[59] Seurynck-Servoss, S.L., M.T. Dohm, and A.E. Barron, *Effects of including an N-terminal insertion region and arginine-mimetic side chains in helical peptoid analogues of lung surfactant protein B.* Biochemistry, 2006. 45(39): p. 11809-18.

[60] Revak, S.D., et al., *Efficacy of synthetic peptide-containing surfactant in the treatment of respiratory distress syndrome in preterm infant rhesus monkeys.* Pediatr Res, 1996. 39(4 Pt 1): p. 715-24.

[61] Lal, M.K. and S.K. Sinha, *Surfactant respiratory therapy using Surfaxin/sinapultide.* Ther Adv Respir Dis, 2008. 2(5): p. 339-44.

[62] Guarnieri, F., et al., *A human surfactant peptide-elastase inhibitor construct as a treatment for emphysema.* Proc Natl Acad Sci U S A, 2010. 107(23): p. 10661-6.

[63] Li, Z., et al., *Oxidized {alpha}1-antitrypsin stimulates the release of monocyte chemotactic protein-1 from lung epithelial cells: potential role in emphysema.* Am J Physiol Lung Cell Mol Physiol, 2009. 297(2): p. L388-400.

[64] Bergin, D.A., et al., *alpha-1 Antitrypsin regulates human neutrophil chemotaxis induced by soluble immune complexes and IL-8.* J Clin Invest, 2010. 120(12): p. 4236-50.

[65] Wiemer, A.J., et al., *Calpain inhibition impairs TNF-alpha-mediated neutrophil adhesion, arrest and oxidative burst.* Mol Immunol, 2010. 47(4): p. 894-902.

[66] Al-Omari, M., et al., *The acute phase protein, alpha1-antitrypsin, inhibits neutrophil calpain I and induces random migration.* Mol Med, 2011.

[67] Lucas, S.D., et al., *Targeting COPD: Advances on low-molecular-weight inhibitors of human neutrophil elastase.* Med Res Rev, 2011.

[68] Luffer-Atlas, D., et al., *Orally active inhibitors of human leukocyte elastase. III. Identification and characterization of metabolites of L-694,458 by liquid chromatography-tandem mass spectrometry.* Drug Metab Dispos, 1997. 25(8): p. 940-52.

[69] Macdonald, S.J., et al., *Discovery of further pyrrolidine trans-lactams as inhibitors of human neutrophil elastase (HNE) with potential as development candidates and the crystal structure of HNE complexed with an inhibitor (GW475151).* J Med Chem, 2002. 45(18): p. 3878-90.

5

Combined Pulmonary Fibrosis and Emphysema (CPFE)

Keisaku Fujimoto[1] and Yoshiaki Kitaguchi[2]
[1]*Department of Clinical Laboratory Sciences, Shinshu University School of Health Sciences.*
[2]*1st Department of Internal Medicine, Shinshu University School of Medicine. Nagano, Japan*

1. Introduction

Combined pulmonary fibrosis and emphysema (CPFE) is one of smoking-related lung diseases.

Emphysema is characterized by the permanent abnormal enlargement of airspaces distal to the terminal bronchioles, accompanied by destruction of their walls. The characteristics of emphysema do not, by definition, include thickening of the alveolar septa and fibrosis. However, coincidental idiopathic pulmonary fibrosis (IPF) and emphysema was firstly reported in 1990 by Wiggins et al (Wiggins J, et al., 1990) in London. Smoking-related interstitial lung diseases (SRILD) include desquamative interstitial pneumonia (DIP), respiratory bronchiolitis-related interstitial lung disease (RB-ILD), pulmonary Langerhans' cell histiocytosis (LCH) and idiopathic pulmonary fibrosis (IPF) (Ryu JH, et al., 2001). Tobacco smoking is also major course of emphysema and chronic obstructive pulmonary disease (COPD). Smoking is a common risk factor for both emphysema and pulmonary fibrosis. Recently, the occurrence of both emphysema and pulmonary fibrosis in the same patient has received increased attention as the syndrome of combined pulmonary fibrosis and emphysema (CPFE) (Cottin V, et al., 2005). It has been demonstrated that CPFE syndrome is not rare because on a series of 110 patients with IPF, 28% of them with at least 10% of the lung affected with emphysema, and thus are considered to have CPFE (Mejia M, et al., 2009).

2. Clinical characteristics of CPFE

In Japan Hiwatari *et al* (Hiwatari N, et al., 1993) reported nine patients with pulmonary emphysema and IPF among 152 pulmonary emphysema patients in 1993. Those patients were all men and heavy smokers. Odani *et al* (Odani K, et al., 2004) reported 31 patients combined with pulmonary emphysema and IPF among 14900 patients who underwent chest CT from January 1996 to March 2001 at Kochi Medical School Hospital in Japan. The CT of all patients showed the coexistence of emphysema with upper lung field predominance and diffuse parenchymal lung disease with significant pulmonary fibrosis predominantly in the lower lung fields (Figure 1). Centriacinar emphysema was present in 24 of the 31 (77%)

patients and paraseptal emphysema in 11 of 31 patients (35%). Honeycombing, which is one of the most common findings of usual interstitial pneumonia, was present in 24 of the 31 patients (77%). In 2005 Cottin *et al* (Cottin V, et al., 2005) conducted a retrospective study of 61 patients with CPFE and characterized this association as a distinct entity. They reported that sixty patients were male, dyspnea on exertion was present in all patients, basal crackles were found in 87% and finger clubbing in 43%. Pulmonary function tests showed preserved lung volumes and strongly impaired lung diffusing capacity for carbon monoxide (DLCO). They showed that pulmonary hypertension was frequent in patients with CPFE with 47% of patients with estimated systolic right ventricular pressure ≧45 mmHg at echocardiography and the 5-yr probability of survival was 25% in patients with pulmonary hypertension compared with 75% in those without pulmonary hypertension at diagnosis (Figure 2). They also confirmed these findings by right heart catheterization on a retrospective multicenter study and concluded that the patients with CPFE and pulmonary hypertension have a dismal prognosis despite moderately altered lung volume and flows (Cottin V, et al., 2010). The risk of developing pulmonary hypertension is much higher in CPFE than in IPF without emphysema (Mejia M, et al., 2009). Pulmonary hypertension was a critical determinant of the prognosis.

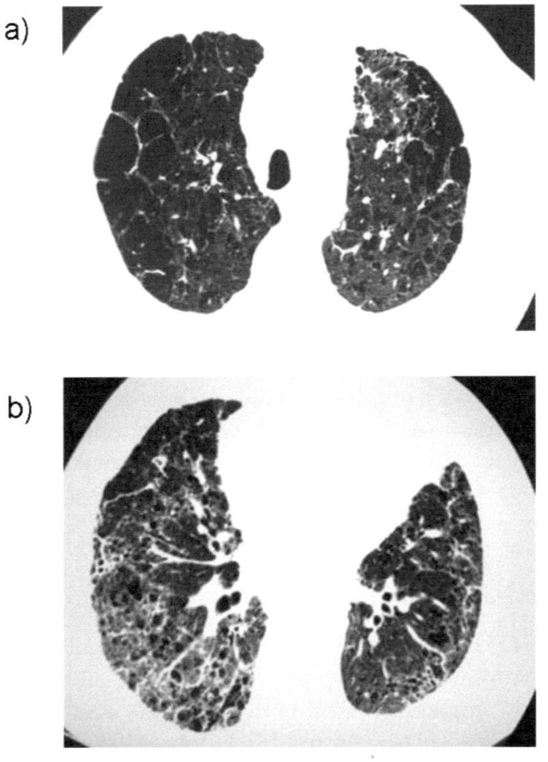

Fig. 1. Imaging in a 66-year-old male with combined pulmonary fibrosis and emphysema (CPFE). Chest high-resolution computed tomography of the bilateral upper lung fields (a) shows centriaciner + paraseptal emphysema with thick walled bulla and of the bilateral lower lung fields (b) shows reticular opacities and traction bronchiectasis.

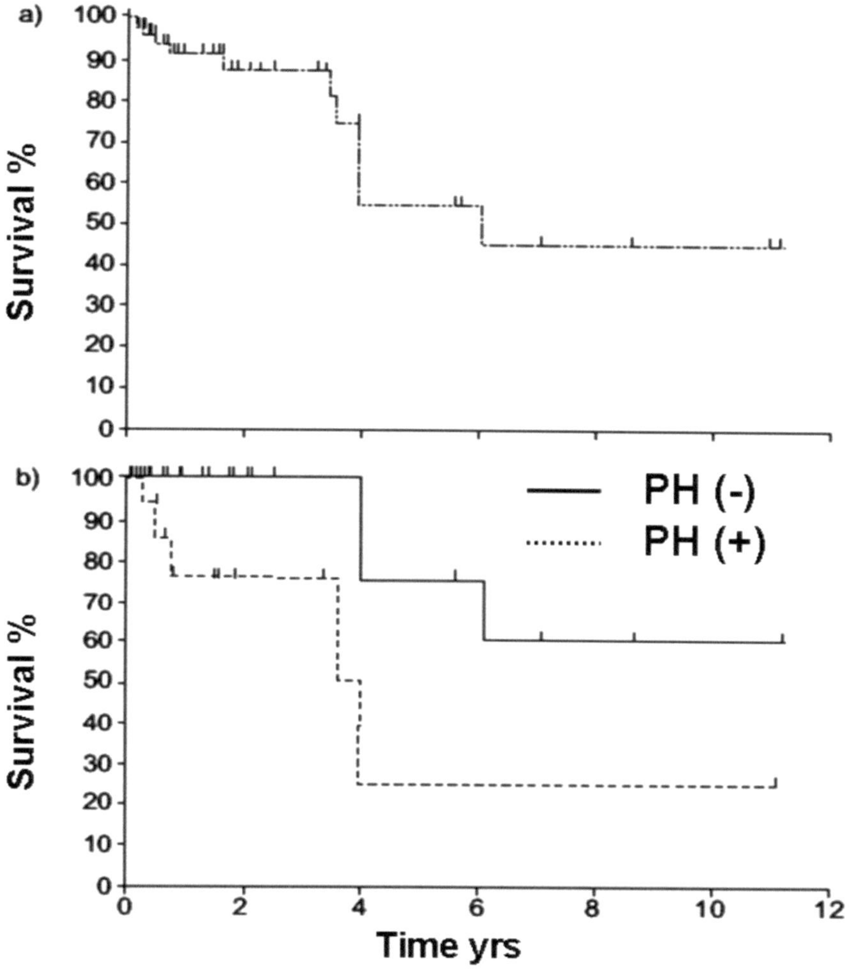

Fig. 2. Total survival of patients with combined pulmonary fibrosis and emphysema (CPFE) (a); 5-yr survival was 55%. Survival for subjects with CPFE stratified on the basis of pulmonary hypertension (PH) (b); 5-yr survival was significantly less in patients with pulmonary hypertension (25%) compared with those without pulmonary hypertension (75%) at diagnosis.

We retrospectively examined the clinical characteristics of 47 patients with CPFE based on the findings of chest HRCT consecutively recruited from outpatients attending Shinshu University Hospital between October 2004 and June 2007 (Kitaguchi Y, et al., 2010). The clinical characteristics of CPFE patients were compared with those of emphysema-dominant COPD patients without parenchymal lung disease (COPD without fibrosis). Forty-six of the 47 CPFE patients were male. Paraseptal emphysema was particularly common in the CPFE group, although centriacinar was dominant in the COPD without fibrosis (Table 1). All CPFE patients showed the coexistence of emphysema with upper lung fields predominance and diffuse parenchymal lung disease with significant pulmonary fibrosis with lower lung fields predominance. Honeycombing, ground-glass opacities and reticular opacities were present in 75.6%, 62.2% and 84.4% of CPFE patients, respectively. Thick-walled bullae were characteristic in CPFE and observed in more than one half of the CPFE patients.

Twenty-seven of the 47 CPFE patients (57.4%) showed a FEV_1/FVC ratio within the normal range and the other patients showed milder airflow limitation, although the presence of severe emphysema (Table 2, 3). All CPFE patients showed lower lung volume and DLCO than the patients with COPD without fibrosis as previously reported. Desaturation during 6-min walking test in CPFE patients tended to be more severe than in COPD without fibrosis patients, if the level of FEV_1 or 6-minute walking distance was equal (Figure 3). These findings suggest that CPFE patients show severe dyspnea and severe hypoxemia on effort in spite of subnormal spirometry findings.

	CPFE	COPD
LAA score	13.2±0.9**	18.9±0.7
Upper lobe	5.6±0.3**	6.7±0.2
Middle lobe	4.3±0.3**	6.2±0.2
Lower lobe	3.3±0.4**	5.9±0.3
Emphysema type		
centriacinar, %	11 (24.4%)**	49 (59.8%)
panacinar+centriacinar, %	7 (15.6%)*	26 (31.7%)
paraseptal, %	15 (33.3%)**	7 (8.5%)
paraseptal+centriacinar, %	12 (26.7%)**	0 (0.0%)
IP distribution		
Upper lobe	8 (17.0%)	
Middle lobe	18 (38.3%)	
Lower lobe	47 (100.0%)	
IP pattern		
Thick-walled bulla, n (%)	26 (57.8%)	
honeycombing, n (%)	34 (75.6%)	
reticular opacity, n (%)	38 (84.4%)	
ground glass opacity, n (%)	28 (62.2%)	
consolidation, n (%)	6 (13.3%)	
traction bronchiectasis, n (%)	18 (40.0%)	
peribronchovascular thickening, n (%)	4 (8.9%)	
architectural distortion, n (%)	7 (15.6%)	

Values are the mean±SEM · *p<0.05 and **p<0.01 vs. COPD.

Table 1. Chest HRCT findings in patients with combined pulmonary fibrosis and emphysema (CPFE, n=47) and emphysema dominant COPD without fibrosis (COPD, n=82).

	CPFE	COPD
number	47	82
Sex, female/male	1/46	8/74
Body mass index, kg/m^2	22.9±0.4**	20.5±0.3
Smoking history, packs • year	58.7±4.4	59.4±3.0
Non-COPD	27 (57.4%)	0 (0.0%)
COPD	20 (42.6%)	82 (100.0%)
Stage I	8 (17.0%)	8 (9.8%)
Stage II	8 (17.0%)**	34 (41.5%)
Stage III	4 (8.5%)**	30 (36.6%)
Stage IV	0 (0.0%)*	10 (12.2%)
Complication of lung cancer、n (%)	22 (46.8%)**	6 (7.3%)
squamous cell carcinoma	12 (54.5%)**	3 (50.0%)
small cell carcinoma	2 (9.1%)	0 (0.0%)
adenocarcinoma	7 (31.8%)	3 (50.0%)
LCNEC	1 (4.5%)	0 (0.0%)

n (%), Values are the mean±SEM · *p<0.05 and **p<0.01 vs. COPD.

Table 2. Clinical characteristics in patients with combined pulmonary fibrosis and emphysema (CPFE) and emphysema dominant COPD without fibrosis (COPD).

	CPFE	COPD
%VC, %	94.7±3.5	96.6±2.4
FEV1, % of pred.	79.0±3.1**	54.7±2.7
FEV1/FVC, %	71.8±2.0**	48.0±1.2
FRC, % of pred.	89.9±5.8**	112.5±2.7
RV, % of pred.	114.7±10.3**	181.7±5.5
RV/TLC, %	37.3±1.9**	50.5±1.1
%DLco, %	39.6±2.5**	57.7±2.2
PaO_2, torr	68.6±2.3	70.0±1.3
$PaCO_2$, torr	39.3±0.9	40.5±0.6
α1-AT, mg/dl	153±15	190±38
CRP, mg/dl	1.1±0.3	0.5±0.1
KL-6, U/ml	1058±166	-

Values are the mean±SEM · **p<0.01 vs. COPD.

Table 3. Pulmonary function tests and laboratory data in patients with combined pulmonary fibrosis and emphysema (CPFE, n=47) and emphysema dominant COPD without fibrosis (COPD, n=82).

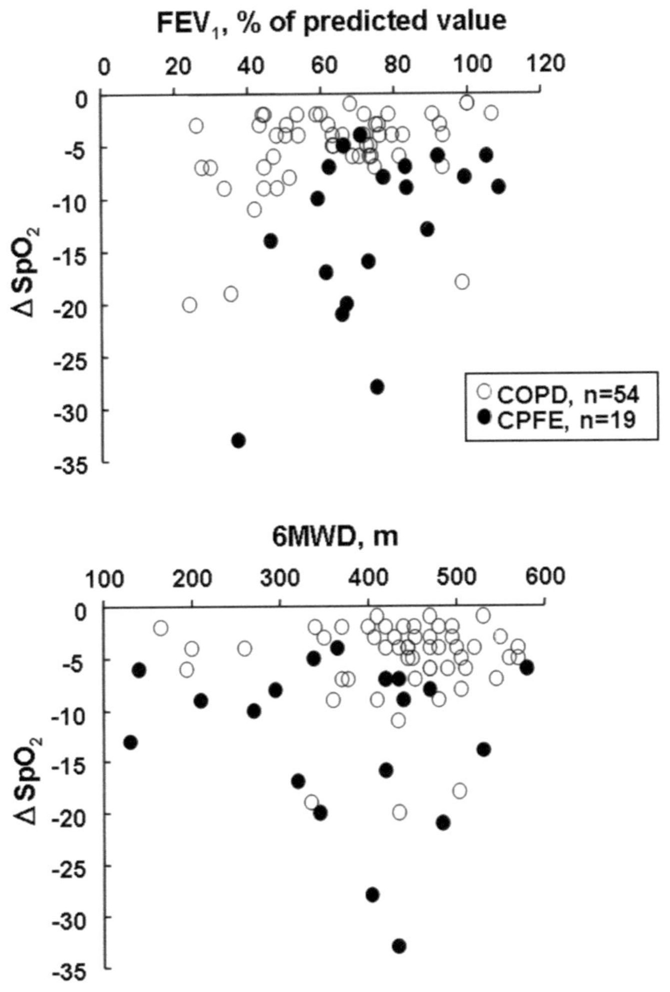

Fig. 3. Relationship between ΔSpO_2 during a 6-minute walking test and FEV_1 or 6 minute-walking distance (6MWD) in patients with combined pulmonary fibrosis and emphysema (CPFE) and emphysema dominant COPD without fibrosis (COPD).

3. Higher incidence of lung cancer

In the series of our retrospective study, twenty-two of the 47 CPFE patients (46.8%) had lung cancer whereas only 7.3% of the patients with COPD without fibrosis had (Table 2) (Kitaguchi Y, et al., 2010). There were no significant differences in histological type of cancer between CPFE and COPD without fibrosis group. Odani *et al* (Odani K, et al., 2004) also reported higher incidence of lung cancer and 42% (13 patients) of CPFE were complicated lung cancer as well as our report and squamous cell carcinoma was the most common histological type. On the other hand, Nakayama et al reported that 18 of 127 patients with COPD (14%) were complicated with lung cancer in Japan (Nakayama M, et al., 2003).

According to a clinical study of IPF based on autopsy studies in elderly patients performed in Japan, lung cancer developed in approximately 23% of the IPF patients (Araki T, et al., 2003). Therefore, the complicated ratio of lung cancer might be higher in CPFE patients than in COPD and IPF patients. However, the evidence is poor because of retrospective study and a single institution study may have some selection bias. Further investigations are needed to clarify whether CPFE is an independent risk factor for lung cancer, its role in susceptibility to lung cancer.

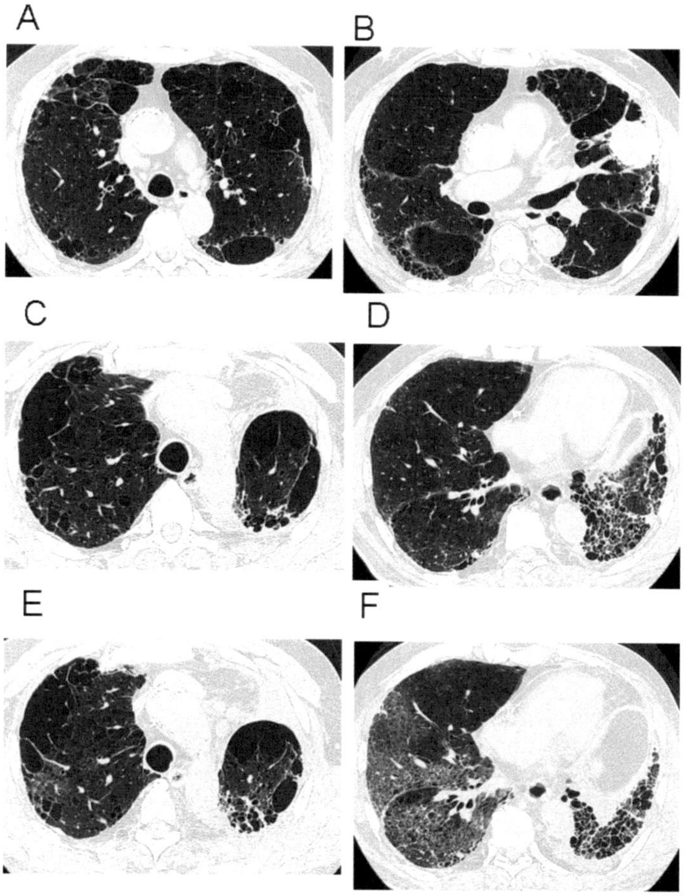

Fig. 4. Imaging in a 78-year-old male with CPFE complicated with lung cancer (squamous cell carcinoma) in the left lung S4. Chest HRCT images before left upper lobectomy (A, B) and after upper lobectomy (C, D). Two months later, the patients developed exacerbation of interstitial pneumonia, new diffuse bilateral ground-glass opacities superimposed on a background of reticular opacities and honeycombing with basal and peripheral predominance (E, F).

When the patients with CPFE are complicated with lung cancer, it may have a profound influence on their prognosis because of poor operability and difficulties in chemotherapy. Usui et al (Usui K, et al., 2011) retrospectively reviewed the data for 1143 patients with lung cancer. CPFE, emphysema and fibrosis were identified in 8.9%, 35.3% and 1.3% patients with lung cancer, retrospectively. The median overall survival of CPFE patients was significantly less than that of normal patients or that of patients with emphysema alone. Of interest, 76% of lung cancers in patients with CPFE were diagnosed at an advanced stage. Also, fatal severe acute lung injury occurred more frequently (19.8%) in CPFE, irrespective of the treatment modality. Especially, postoperative lung injury occurred in nine of 33 patients with CPFE. Therefore, the presence of CPFE may be higher risk for postoperative lung injury as well as the presence of interstitial lung disease (Chiyo M, et al., 2003). Figure 4 shows imaging in a 78-year-old male with CPFE complicated with lung cancer (squamous cell carcinoma) in the segment 4 of left lung admitted to our hospital. He was underwent left upper lobectomy for lung cancer. However, two months later, he developed severe exacerbation of interstitial pneumonia, and dies due to respiratory failure.

4. Pathogenesis

Little is known about the pathogenesis of CPFE. Concerning with parenchymal lung disease in CPFE, usual interstitial pneumonia (UIP) has been the most common histopathological finding, and there are no differences in histological findings from IPF. IPF and pulmonary emphysema have distinct clinical and pathological characteristics, and have been considered to be separate disorders. In spite of such differences, animal experiments have suggested that the same lung injury might result in either fibrosis or emphysema. Connective tissue synthesis during the healing phase may be the critical determinant (Niewoehner DE, et al., 1982). Hoyle *et al.* (Hoyle GW, et al., 1999) reported that the overexpression of platelet-derived growth factor-B induced both emphysema and fibrotic lung disease in the developing and adult lung of transgenic mice. It has been also shown that the overexpression of TNF-alpha driven by the surfactant protein C promoter (Lundblad LK, et al., 2005), IL-13 (Fulkerson PC, et al., 2006), and transforming growth factor-beta 1 (Lee CG, et al., 2006) in transgenic mice induces pathological changes consistent with both emphysema and pulmonary fibrosis. These pathological changes might represent an experimental animal model of CPFE. The tissue effects of these factors might depend on the balance of apoptosis, proteolysis and fibrosis and might regulate the degree of emphysema and/or fibrosis in the injured lung. It has been recently reported a 32-year-old women, never smokers, with CPFE and her daughter at 3 months of age showed having fibrosing interstitial pneumonia, and both the mother and daughter had a mutation of the surfactant protein-C (SFTPC) gene (Cottin V, et al., 2011). It is suggested that an individual's genetic background may predispose some smokers to the development of CPFE. Further studies are needed to elucidate these phenomena.

5. Conclusion

CPFE patients had some different clinical characteristics in comparison with emphysema and interstitial lung disease and should be included as a smoking-related lung disease. The patients with CPFE show severe dyspnea, unexpected subnormal spirometry findings, severely impaired DLCO, hypoxemia at exercise, characteristic imaging feature, and a high probability of severe pulmonary hypertension and lung cancer. A strict follow-up is therefore required because of higher rate of complicated pulmonary hypertension and lung cancer and acute exacerbation may occur after lung surgery in CPFE. HRCT plays an important role in diagnose CPFE and evaluating the occurrence of lung cancer and an acute exacerbation of CPFE. CPFE syndrome is an important entity and is a matter of growing interest by respiratory clinicians.

6. References

Araki T, Katsura H, Sawabe M, Kida K. A clinical study of idiopathic pulmonary fibrosis based on autopsy studies in elderly patients. *Intern. Med.* 2003; 42: 483-9.

Chiyo M, Sekine Y, Iwata T et al. Impact of interstitial lung disease on surgical morbidity and mortality for lung cancer: analyses of short-term and long-term outcome. J Thorac Cardiovasc Surg 2003; 126: 1141-6.

Cottin V, Le Pavec J, Prevot G, et al. Pulmonary hypertention in patients with combined pulmonary fibrosis and emphysema syndrome. Eur Respir J 2010; 35: 105-111.

Cottin V, Nunes H, Brillet PY, et al. Combined pulmonary fibrosis and emphysema: a distinct underrecognised entity. Eur Respir J 2005 26: 586-93.

Cottin V, Reix P, Khouatra C, et al. Combined pulmonary fibrosis and emphysema syndrome associated with familial SFTPC mutation. Thorax , 2011.

Fulkerson PC, Fischetti CA, Hassman LM *et al.* Persistent effects induced by IL-13 in the lung. *Am. J.Respir.CellMol.Biol.* 2006; 35: 337–46.

Hiwatari N, Shimura S, Takishima T. Pulmonary emphysema followed by pulmonary fibrosis of undetermined cause. *Respiration* 1993; 60: 354-8.

Hoyle GW, Li J, Finkelstein JB *et al.* Emphysematous lesions, inflammation, and fibrosis in the lungs of transgenic mice overexpressing platelet-derived growth factor. *Am. J. Pathol.* 1999; 154: 1763–75.

Kitaguchi Y, Fujimoto K, Hanaoka M, et al. Clinical characteristics of combined pulmonary fibrosis and emphysema. Respirology 2010 15: 265-71.

Lee CG, Cho S, Homer RJ *et al.* Genetic control of transforming growth factor-beta1-induced emphysema and fibrosis in the murine lung. *Proc. Am. Thorac. Soc.* 2006; 3: 476–7.

Lundblad LK, Thompson-Figueroa J, Leclair T *et al.* Tumor necrosis factor-alpha overexpression in lung disease: a single cause behind a complex phenotype. *Am. J. Respir. Crit. CareMed.* 2005; 171: 1363–70.

Mejia M, Carrillo G, Rojas-Serrano J, et al. Idiopathic pulmonary fibrosis and emohysema: decreased survival associated with severe pulmonary arterial hypertension. Chest 2009; 136: 10-15.

Nakayama M, Satoh H, Sekizawa K. Risk of cancers in COPD patients. Chest. 2003; 123: 1775-6.

Niewoehner DE, Hoidal JR. Lung fibrosis and emphysema: divergent responses to a common injury? *Science* 1982; 217: 359–60.

Odani K, Murata Y, Yoshida S. Computed Tomographic Evaluation in the Cases of Coexistence of Pulmonary Emphysema with Idiopathic Pulmonary Fibrosis. *Danso Eizo kenkyukai Zasshi* (Japanese Journal of Tomography) 2004; 31: 25-9.

Ryu JH, Colby TV, Hartman TE, Vassallo R. Smoking-related interstitial lung diseases: a concise review. Eur Respir J 2001 17: 122-32.

Usui K, Tanai C, Tanaka Y, et al. The prevalence of pulmonary fibrosis combined with emphysema in patients with lung cancer. Respirology 2011; 16: 326-331.

Wiggins J, Strickland B, Turner-Warwick M. Combined cryptogenic fibrosing alveolitis and emphysema: the value of high resolution computed tomography in assessment. Respir Med 1990; 84: 365-369.

6

Endoscopic Lung Volume Reduction

Daniela Gompelmann and Felix J.F. Herth
University of Heidelberg, Thoraxklinik,
Pneumology and Respiratory Care Medicine, Thoraxklinik, Heidelberg
Germany

1. Introduction

Chronic obstructive pulmonary disease (COPD) that presents a growing cause for mortality worldwide [1, 2] is characterized by chronic bronchitis, obstructive bronchiolitis and emphysema. The most important etiologic factor is cigarette smoking, but occupational and environmental dusts as well as genetic factors contribute to COPD developing. The exposure to these noxious inhaled agents lead to abnormal pathogenic reactions like a permanent airway inflammation, imbalance between proteinases and antiproteinases, impairment of elastin repair and increased oxidative stress with subsequent lung parenchyma destruction [3]. The progressive permanent enlargement of airspaces distal to terminal bronchioles results in a decrease in lung elastic recoil, air trapping and hyperinflation, thus leading to airflow limitation and increased residual volume. These alterations of respiratory mechanics cause the symptoms of dyspnoea, limited exercise capacitiy and reduced quality of life. Therapeutic recommendations for COPD consisting of bronchodilators, glucocorticosteroids, long term oxygen therapy and rehabilitation are common insufficient in advanced COPD [4]. Therefore, surgical treatments like Lung Volume Reduction Surgery (LVRS) and lung transplantation should be considered in advanced disease. The resection of emphysematous lung tissue results in improvement of lung elastic recoil with subsequent increased expiratory flow. Furthermore, the reduction of hyperinflation allows the diaphragm to function more effectively and increases the global inspiratory muscle strength [5].

Already in the 1950s, the first lung volume reduction surgery has been performed to achieve lung volume reduction with subsequent improvement of respiratory mechanics leading to decreased breathlessness on exertion and increased exercise capacity. Although a physiological improvement could be observed, the surgical treatment did not attract attention due to high perioperative mortality [6]. Just in the 1990s the surgical treatment was reintroduced and the positive results have been confirmed in several trials [7-10]. The most known trial related to LVRS is the multicenter "National Emphysema Treatment Trial" (NETT) [10] comparing the surgical treatment to standard medical care in 1.218 patients with severe emphysema. The results of NETT showed that patients with predominantly upper lobe emphysema experienced significant improvement in clinical outcome measurements. However, the 90-day mortality rate in the surgery group was 7.9% and thus significant higher than in the medical-therapy group. Particularly, in patients with non upper lobe predominant emphysema and poor lung function, a high mortality could be observed. Therefore, different bronchoscopic approaches have been developed imitating the LVRS but with less morbidity and mortality.

Until now, there are various techniques of Endoscopic Lung VolumeReduction (ELVR) extending the therapeutic strategies in patients withsevere emphysema. In general, reversible blocking techniques and irreversible, non-blocking techniques can be distinguished. The application of these different techniques is dependent on the emphysema distribution and degree of collateral ventilation. Therefore, an accurate patient selection has great importance.

2. Reversible, blocking techniques

The first and most known method of endoscopic lung volume reduction is the implantation of valves in targeted most destroyed lung compartments in patients with heterogeneous emphysema [11]. These blocking devices allow the air to be expelled during expiration but prevent the air entering the target lobe during inspiration and so facilitating atelectasis to achieve lung volume reduction. Two different valves are available: endobronchial valves (EBV, Zephyr ®, Pulmonx, Inc., Palo Alto, Calif., USA) and intrabronchial valves (IBV, Spiration®, Olympus Medical Co., Tokio, Japan).

2.1 Implantation technique

The endobronchial (figure 1) and intrabronchial valves (figure 2) only differentiate in shape, but the implantation technique and their functional principle is very similar. The endobronchial valves consist of a cylindrical nitinol framework, whereas the intrabonchial valves have got an umbrella shaped nitinol skeleton. Both valves are covered by a silicone membrane. Endobronchial valves are available in two different sizes, intrabronchial valves in three different sizes. Prior to valve implantation, the diameter of the bronchus that is considered to be blocked by the valves is estimated by using the measurement wings of the delivery system or a special balloon catheter. Afterwards, the appropriately sized valves are preloaded in a delivery catheter that can be introduced through a 2.8 mm or larger working channel of a standard flexible bronchoscope. The catheter is placed in the airway of the target lobe and by retracting the sheath, the valve can be deployed easily that expanded against the bronchial wall. The procedure can be performed under general anesthesia as well as under conscious sedation and takes generally 10 to 30 minutes depending on the number of valves that are placed.

2.2 Endobronchial valves (EBV)

The first published trials related to endoscopic lung volume reduction by valves were about the implantation of EBV in patients with severe heterogeneous emphysema by Toma et al. and Snell et al. in 2003 [12; 13]. Since then, several series have been published [14; 15]. The biggest and most noted trail however is the "Endobronchial Valve for Emphysema Palliation Trial" (VENT) that has been published by Sciurba et al. in 2007 [16]. In this prospective trial, 321 patients with severe emphysema were randomly assigned in a 2:1 ratio to receive endobronchial valve treatment or standard medical care. 6 months following the treatment, the results referring to the lung function test revealed a mean between group-difference of 6.8% in FEV_1.

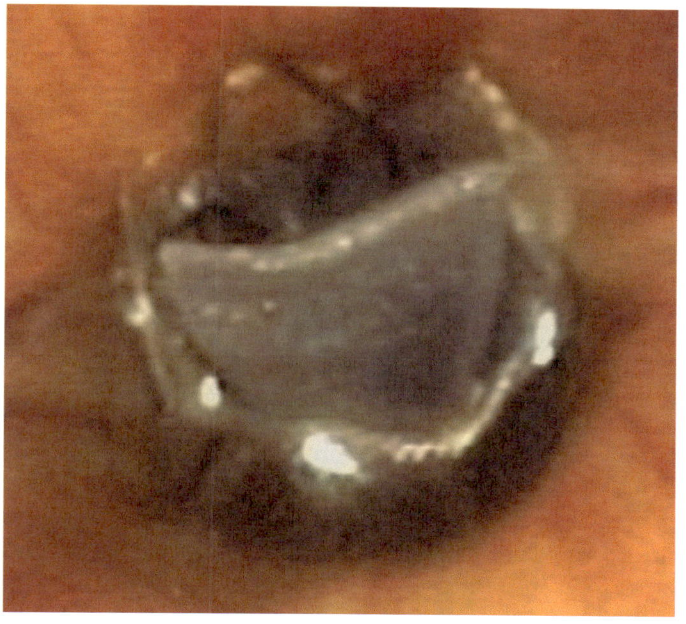

Fig. 1. Endobronchial valve.

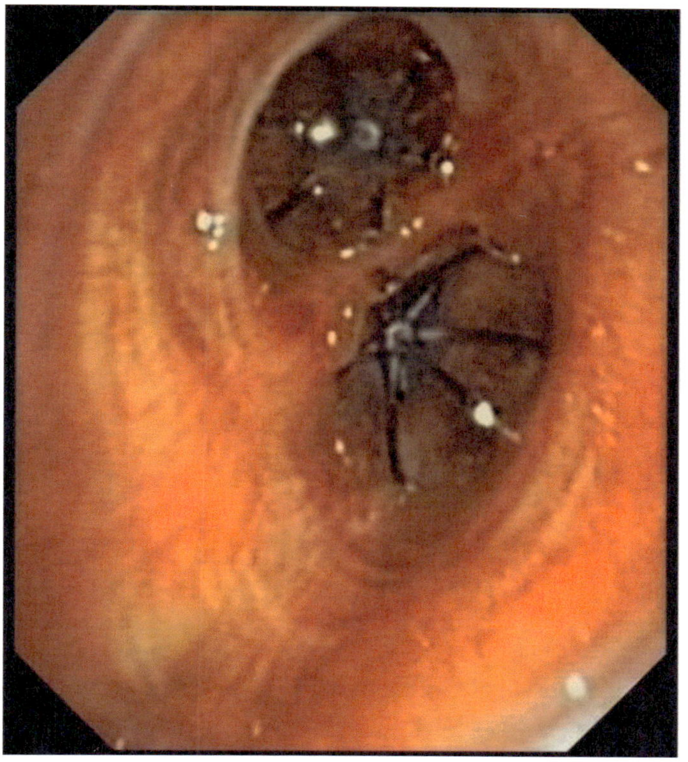

Fig. 2. Intrabronchial valve.

Furthermore, a mean between-group difference of 5.8% in the 6-minute-walk distance could be detected. Among the patients who received EBV, there was a greater reduction in the lung volume of the target lobe measured by high-resolution computed tomography (HRCT). At 12 months, the complication rate was 10.3% in the EBV group versus 4.2% in the control group. Some predictive characteristics were observed in sub analysis of this study. The beneficial effects were greatest in patients with presence of high heterogeneity of their emphysema distribution and an accurate lobar exclusion by the valves. Furthermore, interlobar fissure integrity that was analyzed as a surrogate for collateral ventilation (CV) in the computed tomography has also been observed as an independent predictor of treatment response. Therefore it is thought that CV is one of the most relevant factors responsible for valve therapy failure. Nowadays, there are two different options to predict the CV and thus the success of valve treatment. On the one hand, fissure integrity can be assessed in the HRCT, on the other hand, a catheter-based endobronchial approach providing quantitatively measurement of collateral resistance has been proposed (figure 3). In one double-blind prospective study in 2010 evaluating the safety and feasibility of this catheter-based system 25 patients with heterogeneous emphysema underwent the endobronchial determination of collateral resistance by using the catheter-based system followed by an EBV treatment [17]. In all patients, the resistance measurement was safely and successfully achieved. A correlation of the measurements with the event of atelectasis after ELVR was found in 90% of the analyzable cases. In a following multicenter study covering patients with severe heterogeneous upper lobe or lower lobe predominant emphysema, the accuracy of this catheter-based system in correctly predicting the target lobe volume reduction was evaluated [18]. Following the CV measurement by using the catheter-based system a complete occlusion of the target lobe by EBV was performed. The target lobe volume reduction after the valve implantation was assessed by HRCT 30 days following the intervention. Out of 80 patients, CV assessment prospectively showed a low CV in 51 patients and a high CV in 29 patients. The accuracy of the catheter-based system in correctly predicting the target lobe volume reduction was found to be 75%. Therefore, this quantitatively measurement of collateral ventilation predicts of whether endoscopic lung volume reduction would be successfully or not.

2.3 Intrabronchial valves (IBV)

There are also several published trials confirming the efficacy of the treatment with intrabronchial valves in patients with heterogeneous emphysema. In most of these studies a bilateral incomplete occlusion of both lobes in patients with upper lobe predominant emphysema was performed to minimize the risk of pneumothorax. The results showed an improvement in health-related quality of life and regional lung volume changes measured by quantitative and qualitative analysis of HRCT [19; 20; 21]. However, in all these studies no significant change in lung function test or 6-minute-walk test could be observed. Therefore, it is thought, that bilateral partial closure leads to redistribution of ventilation but avoid atelectasis with subsequent absence of improvement of these objective clinical outcome measures. To evaluate this hypothesis, a randomized prospective study comparing unilateral complete versus bilateral incomplete endoscopic lung volume reduction by IBV implantation in 20 patients with severe upper lobe predominant emphysema was performed

[22]. The results demonstrated a greater benefit in patients receiving the unilateral endoscopic lung volume reduction with complete occlusion of one lobe. Significant differences were evaluated in FEV_1 (+32.5% vs. +2.5%) as well as in the 6-minute-walk test (+43m vs. -19m). In conclusion, unilateral treatment with complete occlusion appears superior to bilateral incomplete treatment but with higher risk of pneumothorax.

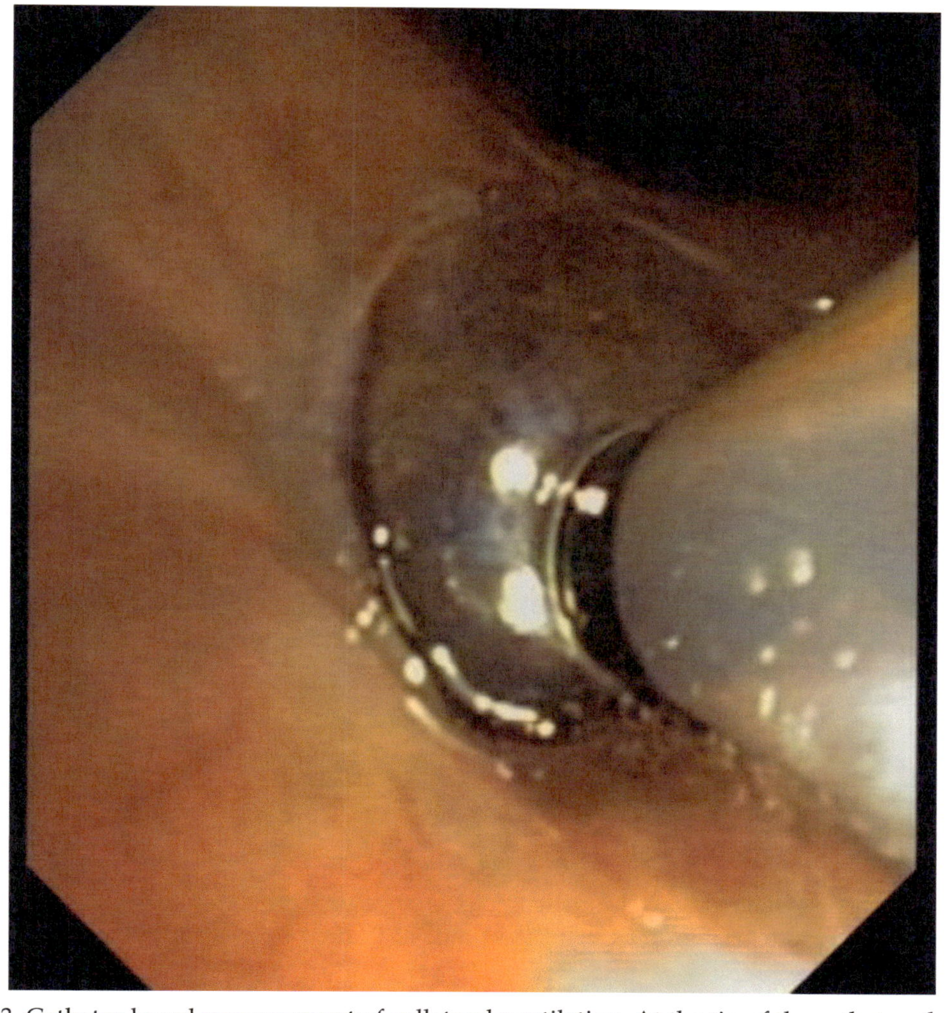

Fig. 3. Catheter-based measurement of collateral ventilation. At the tip of the catheter, there is a balloon, that is be inflated within the airway to isolate the target lobe. The air is directed through the catheter to the console for measurement of air flow and air pressure.

3. Irreversible, non-blocking techniques

Besides the blocking devices, there are various non-blocking techniques for bronchoscopic emphysema therapy. Implantation of lung volume reduction coils, polymeric lung volume reduction, bronchoscopic thermal vapour ablation and creation of airway bypasses can be distinguished. These techniques seem to be independent of collateral ventilation, however these methods are irreversible.

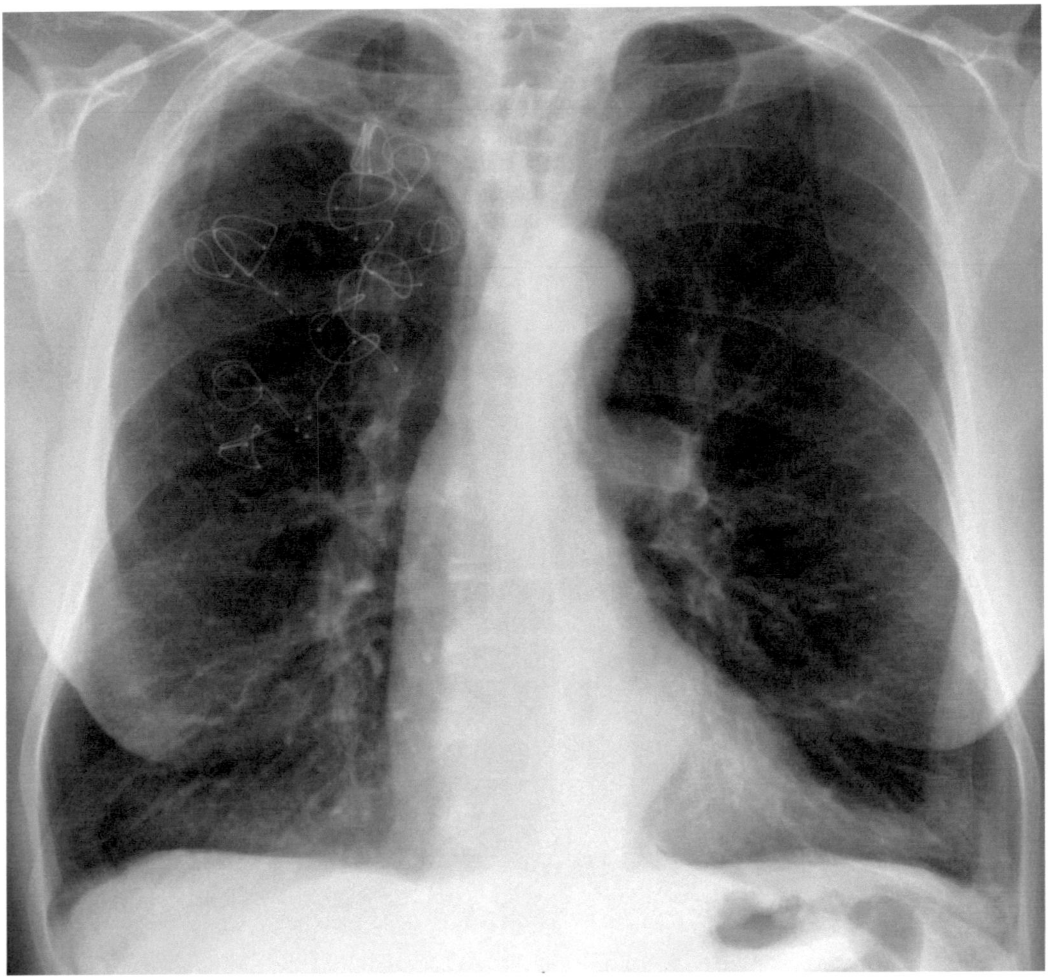

Fig. 4. Chest x-ray following the implantation of lung volume reduction coils in the right upper lobe. In courtesy of Prof. Dr. med. CP Heussel, Thoraxklinik Heidelberg.

3.1 Lung Volume Reduction Coils (LVRC)

One of these non-blocking endoscopic techniques is the implantation of lung volume reduction coils (LVRC, PneumRx, Inc., Mountain View, Calif., USA). These coils consisting of a nitinol wire have got a preformed shape that results in parenchymal compression and thus achieving a lung volume reduction. For implantation, the airway is identified bronchoscopically. Afterwards a low stiffness guidewire is advanced into the airway under fluoroscopic guidance with a distance of 15 mm between the distal end of the guidewire and the pleura. Next, a catheter is passed over the guidewire. Then the guidewire is removed and a straightened LVRC is introduced. As the catheter is pulled back, the coil assumes its preformed shape leading to parenchymal compression. Figure 4 shows a chest x-ray following implantation of coils in the right upper lobe. In a pilot study using coils in heterogeneous as well as in homogeneous emphysema, the patients with predominant heterogeneous disease appeared to show more substantial improvements in pulmonary function, lung volumes, 6 minute walk test and quality of life measures than patients with homogeneous disease [23]. According to these results, a study investigating the efficacy of LVRC treatment in 16 patients with only severe heterogeneous emphysema was performed [24]. 12 patients were treated bilaterally, 4 patients underwent treatment in one lobe. A median of 10 coils per lobe were placed. LVRC treatment in all patients resulted in significant improvements in pulmonary function, exercise capacity and quality of life, with an acceptable safety.

3.2 Polymeric Lung Volume Reduction (PLVR)

Polymeric lung volume reduction (PLVR, Aeris therapeutics, Inc. Woburn, Mass., USA) consists of administration of a foam sealant in the destroyed lung compartment resulting in local inflammatory reaction. This inflammation leads to fibrosis and scarring with subsequent lung volume reduction (figure 5a and 5b). PLVR can be offered to patients with heterogeneous disease, but also patients with homogeneous disease experience improvement after PLVR. However, further trials evaluating the efficacy of PLVR in patients with severe homogeneous emphysema are needed.

The sealant is administered via a special single lumen catheter that is inserted through the working channel of a standard flexible bronchoscope until its tip extends approximately 4 cm from the tip of the scope. During the administration of the sealant, the bronchoscope is maintained in wedge position preventing backflow of the sealant at the airway subsegment. The injection time of the sealant that is prepared in a syringe takes about 10-20 seconds. The bronchoscope should be maintained in wedge position for one minute following delivery to allow complete in situ polymerization. Afterwards, the bronchoscope is repositioned at the next subsegment and the procedure is repeated [25].

The first studies related to PLVR showed encouraging results with beneficial effects in selected patients with heterogeneous emphysema [26; 27] as well as with homogeneous emphysema [28]. Furthermore, a multicenter dose-ranging study revealed, that patients who received high dose treatment with 20 ml per subsegment experienced greater improvement in clinical outcomes than patients with a low dose treatment with 10 ml per subsegment [27]. In these trials, biological reagents were instillated to initiate an inflammatory reaction and a collapse of targeted lung portions, but it then was replaced by synthetic AeriSeal foam that allows a simpler production without blood products.

In one recently published multicenter trial, 25 patients with severe upper lobe predominant emphysema underwent PLVR by using AeriSeal foam [29]. All patients tolerated the treatment without significant adverse events. However, a flu-like reaction following the procedure could be detected in all patients. 24 weeks after the PLVR, physiological and clinical benefits were observed. Furthermore, efficacy responses were better among the patients with COPD GOLD (Global Initiative for Chronic Obstructive Lung Disease) stage III than among patients with COPD GOLD stage IV.

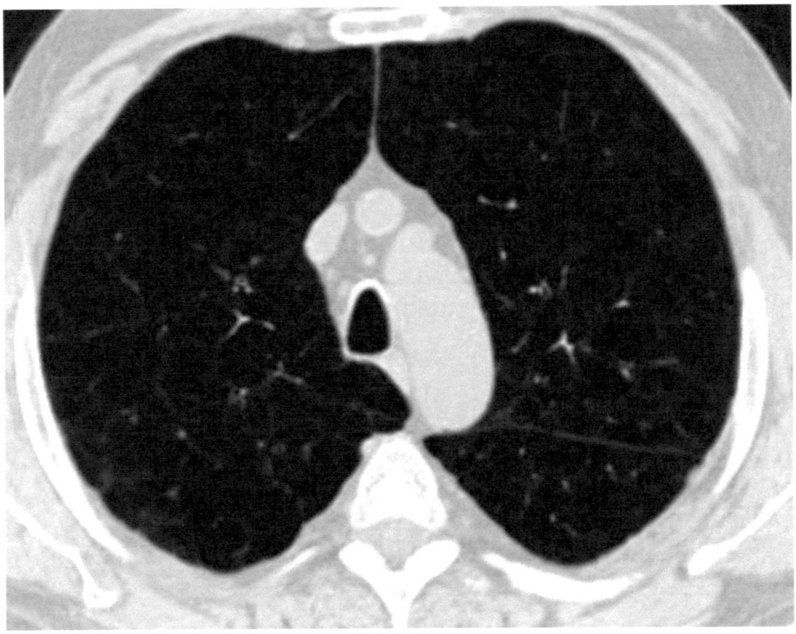

(a)

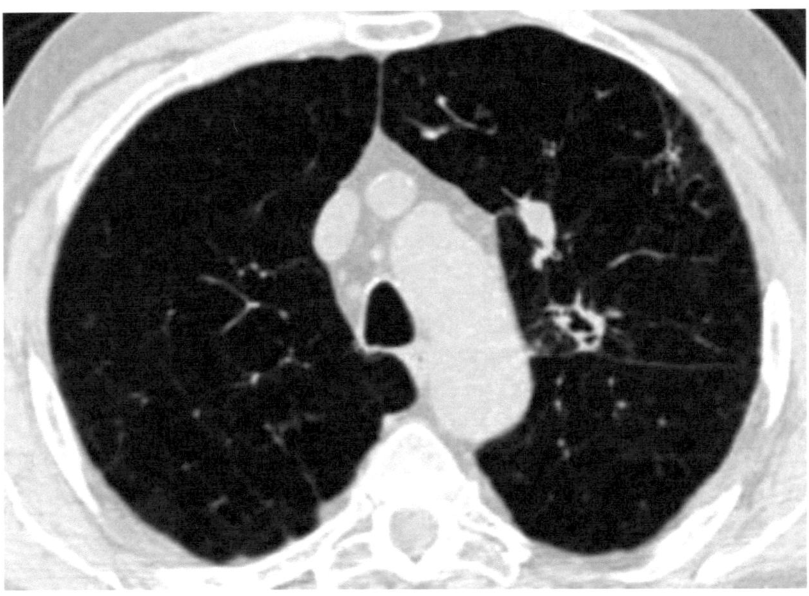

(b)

Fig. 5. Computed tomography acquired prior to polymeric lung volume reduction (a) in the left upper lobe and matched CT scan (b) taken 6 months following the treatment. The shift of the interlobar fissure shows the target lobe volume reduction. In courtesy of Prof. Dr. med. CP Heussel, Thoraxklinik Heidelberg.

3.3 Bronchoscopic Thermal Vapor Ablation (BTVA)

Bronchoscopic thermal vapor ablation (BTVA, Uptake Medical, Seattle, Wash., USA) is an alternative method that is very similar to PLVR. This technique consists of a vapor generator and a special InterVapor catheter used to deliver heated water vapor bronchoscopically to the most destroyed lung regions. The vapor induces an inflammatory reaction with subsequent fibrosis and scarring leading to lung volume reduction (figure 6a and 6b).

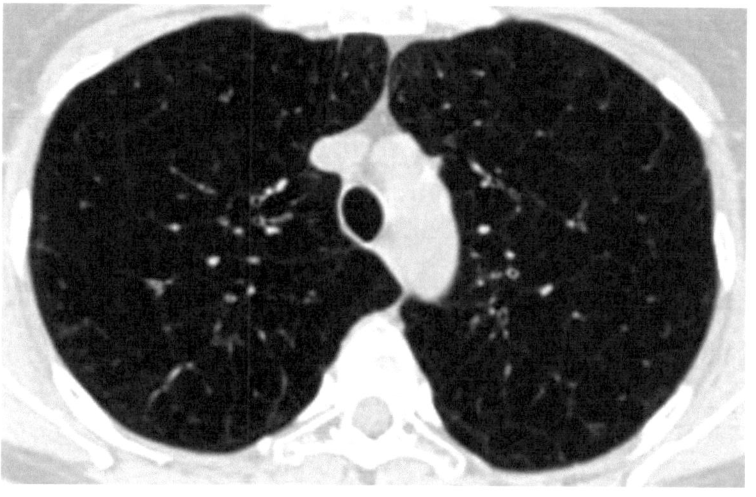

(a)

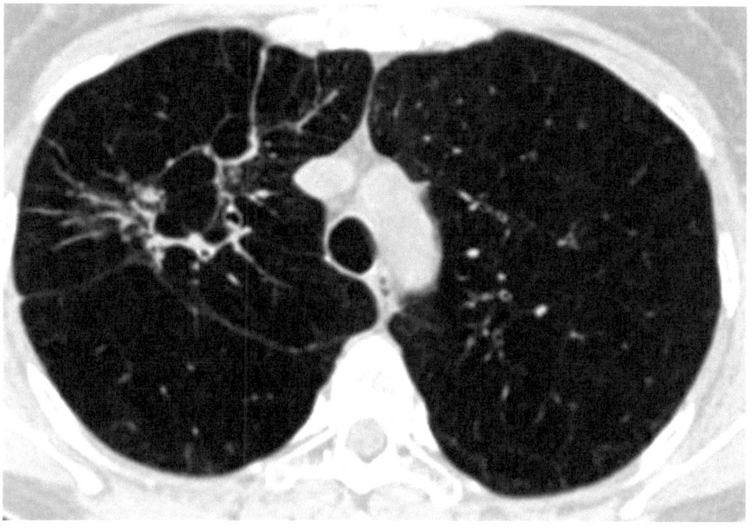

(b)

Fig. 6. Computed tomography taken prior to bronchoscopic thermal vapor ablation (a) in the right upper lobe. 6 months following the treatment a lobar volume reduction can be observed (b). In courtesy of Prof. Dr. med. CP Heussel, Thoraxklinik Heidelberg.

After identifying the target airway bronchoscopically, the InterVapor catheter is introduced through the working channel of the flexible bronchoscope. At the tip of the catheter there is a balloon that can be inflated within the airway so that the target lung region is isolated. Next, a predetermined dose of 125° C heated water vapor is delivered via the special InterVapor catheter.

In a 2009 reported study, 11 patients with heterogeneous emphysema treated by unilateral BTVA confirmed the feasibility and an acceptable safety profile [30]. Furthermore, an improvement of health-related quality of life could be observed. A recently published multinational single arm study evaluated the efficacy of the bronchoscopic thermal vapor ablation in 44 patients with upper lobe predominant emphysema. 24 patients received BTVA in the right upper lobe, 20 patients were treated in the left upper lobe in a single procedure with a target vapor dose of 10 cal/g. During the procedure, no adverse events could be observed. The most common adverse events following the treatment were COPD exacerbations, pneumonia and haemoptysis. 6 months following the treatment, efficacy data showed a 48% reduction of treated lobar volume assessed by HRCT measurement. Furthermore, the patients experienced significant improvement in lung function, exercise capacity and health-related quality of life [31].

3.4 Airway bypass

The creation of extra-anatomic passageways through the normal bronchial wall allowing the trapped air to escape presents a method of endoscopic lung volume reduction in patients with severe homogeneous emphysema (EASE, Broncus Technologies, Inc. Mountain View, USA).

The procedure is performed by using a standard flexible bronchoscope. After identifying the appropriate airway, a Doppler probe is used to confirm the absence of vessels behind the airway wall. Afterwards, the wall is punctured by a transbronchial needle. A balloon catheter is advanced into this hole and the balloon is inflated to enlarge the hole. After repeated confirmation of absence of vessels, a drug-eluting stent (DES) is placed to keep the bypass open over time. The trapped air can escape by bypassing the small airways leading to a lung volume reduction.

In one large prospective, sham-controlled study - EASE trial (Exhale Airway Stents for Emphysema) - 315 patients with severe homogeneous emphysema were subdivided into two groups [32]: only 208 patients out of the 315 patients received the airway bypasses. Immediately post procedure, reductions in lung volume could be evaluated demonstrating proof of concept for airway bypass. However, for the overall group, the initial benefit decreases by 6 months so that at least no sustainable benefit could be recorded with airway bypass in the patients with homogeneous emphysema. The most probable cause for loss of initial benefit is stent occlusion by mucus. Therefore, improvement of durability is required before airway bypasses could be recommend as beneficial therapy.

4. Patient selection

An accurate patient selection is the most important and most difficult issue in the area of endoscopic lung volume reduction. The various approaches require different conditions that must be fulfilled to achieve beneficial outcome. Therefore a treatment algorithm is necessary for identifying the best candidates for the different techniques of endoscopic lung volume reduction.

Patients with severe emphysema have to undergo a screening basic examination programme including lung function testing (spirometry, bodyplethysmography, diffusing capacity measurements), blood gases and exercise tests (6-minute-walk test). Electrocardiogramm, echocardiogram, chest x-ray as well as laboratory testing provide to evaluate patient´s clinical status prior to bronchoscopic intervention. To determine the emphysema distribution as well as fissure integrity, high resolution computed tomography scan at full inspiration and perfusion scan are necessary. Different visual scoring systems e.g. YACTA®, Pulmo® or Volume® can be used for detailed quantitative emphysema analysis. As alternative method to fissure analysis by HRCT, the catheter-based measurement can be performed to evaluate the degree of collateral ventilation.

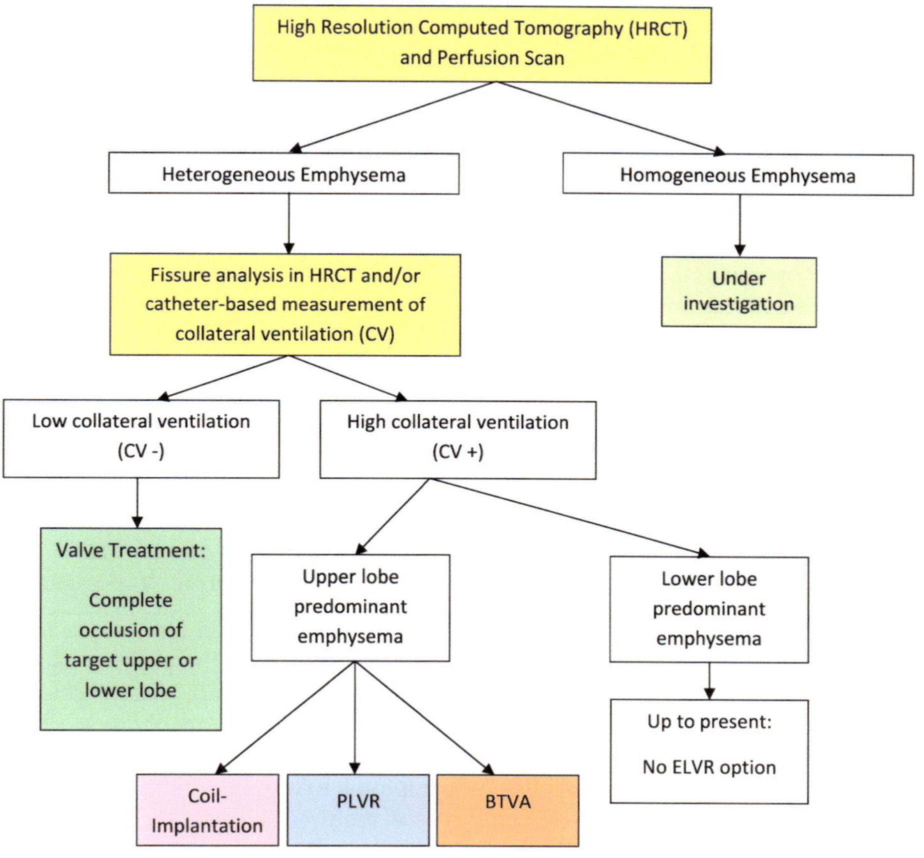

Fig. 7. Patient selection and therapy algorithm.

According to the VENT, following inclusion criteria should be fulfilled: forced expiratory volume in 1 s (FEV_1) < 45%, total lung capacity (TLC) > 100%, residual volume (RV) > 150 %, a partial pressure of arterial carbon dioxide of 50 mm Hg or less, a partial pressure of arterial oxygen of at least 45 mm Hg (without oxygen therapy), a 6-minute-walk distance of > 140 m. Greatest beneficial effects can be observed in patients with a severe hyperinflation with a RV > 200% and a high RV/TLC. Depending on the emphysema distribution and the fissure integrity, the method of endoscopic lung volume reduction is chosen (see figure 1).

5. Complications

5.1 Valve Implantation

The most common adverse event following valve implantation is pneumonia distal the valves despite the valves allow secretion to pass. The VENT revealed a pneumonia rate of 4.2% [16]. In 1/3 of these cases, valve removal was necessary for recovery. In very rare cases, development of bronchiectasis can be observed distal the valves requiring valve removal. Another frequent risk is pneumothorax after valve treatment. Therefore, pneumothorax must be ruled out by chest x-ray 2 hours and 24 h following the intervention. Pneumothorax occurs particularly in patients who experience a great improvement in clinical outcome following valve placement due to a rapid atelectasis. Chest tube drainage is required in some patients with lung collapse. In case of persistent fistula, the removal of one of the implanted valves provides lung expanding and thus sealing fistula. Surgical intervention is only needed to treat fistula that remains persistent despite of adequate chest tube drainage and valve removal. Development of granulation tissue formation that is often associated with bleeding complication is another side effect related to valves due to the pressure of the valves on the mucosa. Cryotherapy is recommended for the treatment of severe granulation tissue formation. New or worsening hypercapnia is another adverse event. Therefore, repeated blood gas analysis following the valve implantation is required. Only in few cases non-invasive ventilation and/or valve removal is necessary. COPD exacerbation, mild haemoptysis, chest pain and valve migration are other anticipated complications to valve treatment.

5.2 Coil Implantation

Side effects rated as possibly related to either the procedure or the device are haemoptysis, dyspnoea, cough, COPD exacerbations, peumonia and chest pain. Pneumothorax can also occur following coil implantation. To minimize risk of pneumothorax, a distance of at least 15 mm to pleura should be kept.

5.3 Polymeric Lung Volume Reduction and Bronchoscopic Thermal Vapor Ablation

The effect of PLVR and BTVA is based on an inflammatory reaction that results in fibrosis, scarring and shrinking. Due to this inflammation, the majority of the patients experience a "flu-like" reaction with dyspnoea, transient fever, pleuritic chest pain, leucocytosis, elevated C-reactive protein and infiltration in chest x-ray. This inflammatory response is self-limiting and resolves within 24-96 h with supportive care. Especially, systemic application of glucocorticosteroids is useful to diminish the symptoms following PLVR. Furthermore, a 7-day course of antibiotic prophylaxis for one week is required in each patient. Other adverse effects following PLVR and BTVA include COPD exacerbation, pneumonia, bronchitis or haemoptysis.

6. Conclusion

Endoscopic lung volume reduction presents an encouraging therapy modality for patients with advanced emphysema. However, efficacy depends strictly on patient selection requiring an appropriate diagnostic and treatment algorithm for identifying the best candidates for each of the various ELVR techniques. Complete lobar occlusion by valve implantation provides an effective option for patients with severe heterogeneous upper lobe or lower lobe predominant emphysema and low collateral ventilation. Irreversible, non-blocking techniques that seem to be independent of collateral ventilation are minimally invasive endoscopic approaches for patients with upper lobe predominant emphysema.

7. References

[1] Lopez AD, Shibuya K, Rao C, Mathers CD, Hansell AL, Held LS, Schmid V, Buist S. Chronic obstructive pulmonary diases: current burden and future projections. Eur Respi J 2006. 27:397-412.

[2] Lopez AD, Mathers CD, Ezzati M, Jamison DT, Murray CJL- Global Burden of Disease and Risk Factors. In: Washington (DC): World Bank. 2006.

[3] Macnee W. Chronic Obstructive Pulmonary Disease: Epidemiology, Physiology and Clinical Evaluation. In Albert RK, Spiro SG, Jett JR (eds): Clinical Respiratory Medicine, Third Edition. Philadelphia: Mosby Elsevier, 2008. 2008. pp 491-516.

[4] Global Initiative for Chronic Obstructive Pulmonary Disease: Global strategy for the diagnosis, management and prevention of COPD.

[5] Marchand E, Gavan-Ramirez G, De Leyn P, Decramer M. Physiological basis of improvement after lung volume reduction surgery for severe emphysema: where are we? Eur Respir J 1999. 13:686-696.

[6] Fessler, HE, Reilly JR, Sugarbaker DJ. Lung Volume Reduction Surgery for Emphysema. N Engl J M 2004. 351:2562-2563.

[7] Cooper JD, Patterson GA, Sundaresan RS et al. Results of 150 consecutive bilateral lung volume reduction procedures in patients with severe emphysema. J Thorac Cardiovasc Surg 1996. 112:1319–1329.

[8] Sciurba FC, Rogers RM, Keenan RJ, Slivka WA, Gorcsan J 3rd, Ferson PF, Holbert JM, Brown ML, Landreneau RJ. Improvement in pulmonary function and elastic recoil after lung-volume reduction surgery for diffuse emphysema. N Engl J Med 1996. 334:1095-1099.

[9] Geddes D, Davies M, Koyama H, Hansell D, Pastorino U, Pepper J, Agent P, Cullinan P, MacNeill SJ, Goldstraw P. Effect of lung-volume-reduction surgery in patients with severe emphysema. N Engl J Med 2000. 343:239-245.

[10] Fishman A, Martinez F, Naunheim K, Piantadosi S, Wise R, Ries A, Weinmann G, Wood DE: A randomized trial comparing lung-volume-reduction surgery with medical therapy for severe emphysema. N Engl J Med 2003; 348: 2059–2073.

[11] Herth FJF, Gompelmann D, Ernst A, Eberhardt R. Endoscopic Lung Volume Reduction. Respiration 2010. 79:5-13.

[12] Toma TP, Hopkinson NS, Hillier J, Hansell DM, Morgan C, Goldstraw PG, Polkey MI, Geddes DM: Bronchoscopic volume reduction with valve implants in patients with severe emphysema. Lancet 2003. 361: 931–933.

[13] Snell GI, Holsworth L, Borrill ZL, Thomson KR, Kalff V, Smith JA, Williams TJ. The potential for bronchoscopic lung volume reduction using bronchial prostheses: a pilot study. Chest 2003; 124: 1073–1080.

[14] Venuta F, de Giacomo T, Rendina EA et al. Bronchoscopic lung-volume reduction with one-way valves in patients with heterogeneous emphysema. Ann Thorac Surg 2005; 79: 411-416; discussion 416-417.

[15] Wan IY, Toma TP, Geddes DM et al. Bronchoscopic lung volume reduction for end-stage emphysema: report on the first 98 patients. Chest 2006; 129: 518-526.

[16] Sciurba FC, Ernst A, Herth FJF, Strange C, Criner GJ, Marquette CH, Kovitz KL, Chiacchierini RP, Goldin J, McLennan G; VENT Study Research Group. A

Randomized Study of Endobronchial Valves for Advanced Emphysema. N Engl J Med 2010; 363(13): 1233-1244.
[17] Gompelmann D, Eberhardt R, Michaud G, Ernst A, Herth FJ. Predicting atelectasis by assessment of collateral ventilation prior to endobronchial lung volume reduction: a feasibility study. Respiration 2010. 80:419-425
[18] Gompelmann D, Eberhardt R, Slebos DJ, Ficker J, Reichenberger F, Schmidt B, Ek L, Herth FJF. Study of the use of Chartis® pulmonary assessment system to optimize subject selection for endobronchial lung volume reduction (ELVR) - Results and subgroup analysis. ERS 2011. Abstract 373.
[19] Wood DE, McKenna RJ, Yusan RD et al. A Multi-Center Trial of an intrabronchial Valve for Treatment of Severe Emphysema. Journal of Thoracic and Cardiovasc Surg 2007. 133:65-73.
[20] Springmeyer SC, Bolliger SC, Waddell TK et al. Treatment of heterogeneous emphysema using the Spiration IBV Valves. Thorac Surg Clinic 2009.
[21] Sterman DH, Mehta AC, Wood De et al. A Multicenter Pilot Study of a Bronchial Valve for the Treatment of Severe Emphysema. Respiration 2010.
[22] Eberhardt R, Gompelmann D, Schuhmann M, Heussel CP, Herth FJF. Unilateral vs. bilateral endoscopic lung volume reduction in patients with severe heterogeneous emphysema: A comparative randomised case study. ERS 2010.
[23] Herth FJF, Eberhardt R, Ernst A: Pilot study of an improved lung volume reduction coil for the treatment of emphysema. Am J Respir Crit Care Med 2009; 179:A6160.
[24] Slebos DJ, Kerstjens HAM, Ernst A, Blaas SH, Gesierich WJ, Herth F. Bronchoscopic lung volume reduction coil treatment of severe heterogeneous emphysema. ERS 2010.
[25] Herth FJ, Eberhardt R, Ingenito EP, Gompelmann D. Assessment of a novel lung sealant for performing endoscopic volume reduction therapy in patients with advanced emphysema. Expert Rev Med Devices 2011. 8:307-312.
[26] Reilly J, Washko G, Pinto-Plata V, Velez E, Kenney L, Berger R, Celli B. Biological lung volume reduction: a new bronchoscopic therapy for advanced emphysema. Chest 2007. 131:1108-1113.
[27] Criner GJ, Pinot-Plata V, Strange C et al. Biologic lung volume reduction in advanced upper lobe emphysema: Phase 2 results. Am J Respir Crit Care 2009. 179:791-798.
[28] Refaely Y, Dransfield M, Kramer MR, Gotfried M, Leeds W, McLennan G, Tewari S, Krasna M, Criner GJ. Biological lung volume reduction therapy for advanced homogeneous emphysema. Eur Respir J 2010. 36:20-27.
[29] Herth FJ, Gompelmann D, Stanzel F, Bonnet R, Behr J, Schmidt B, Magnussen H, Ernst A, Eberhardt R. Treatment of Advanced Emphysema with Emphysematous Lung Sealant (AeriSeal®). Epub ahead of print.
[30] Snell GI, Hopkins P, Wetsall G, Holsworth L, Carle A, Williams TJ. A feasibility and safety study of bronchoscopic thermal vapor ablation: a novel emphysema therapy. Ann Thorac Surg 2009. 88:1993-1998.
[31] Snell G, Herth FJF, Hopkins P, Baker K, Witt Christian, Gotfried MH, Valipour A, Wagner M, Stanzel F, Egan J, Kesten S, Ernst A. Bronchoscopic Thermal Vapor Ablation Therapy in the Management of Heterogeneous Emphysema. Submitted.
[32] Shah P, Slebos DJ, Cardoso PF, Cetti E, Voelker K, Levine B, Russell ME, Goldin J, Brown M, Cooper JD, Sybrecht GW; EASE trial study group. Bronchoscopic lung-volume reduction with Exhale airway stents for emphysema (EASE trial): randomized, sham-controlled, multicentre trial. Lancet 2011. 378:997-1005.

7

Surgical Management of Prolonged Air Leak in Patients with Underlying Emphysema

Boon-Hean Ong[1], Bien-Keem Tan[2] and Chong-Hee Lim[1]
[1]*Department of Cardiothoracic Surgery, National Heart Centre Singapore*
[2]*Department of Plastic, Reconstructive and Aesthetic Surgery, Singapore General Hospital*
Singapore

1. Introduction

Prolonged air leak is one of the most common post-operative complications encountered after thoracic surgical operations involving mobilization or resection of lung parenchyma. Air leak typically manifests as persistent bubbling in a chest tube drainage system, but may also present with increasing subcutaneous emphysema or pneumothorax in a post-operative patient. No universal consensus exist as to the exact duration of air leak which constitutes a prolonged air leak, but it is generally regarded to exist if it is present for more than 5 days(1-4) or 7 days(2, 5-7) after initial surgery. It is an important complication that results in increased length of stay(8-15) and has been associated with other post-operative complications such as pneumonia(12, 14, 16), empyema(9, 10, 16) and ICU re-admission(12).

Patients with emphysema form a significant proportion of patients which will undergo thoracic surgical operations. Chronic smoking and emphysema predisposes an individual to developing a pneumothorax(17, 18) or carcinoma of the lung(19, 20) that may require surgical intervention for treatment. In addition, lung volume reduction surgery plays a role in the management of certain patients with advanced emphysema(21). Conversely, emphysema is regarded as a risk factor for developing prolonged air leak in cases where patients with emphysema require an operation(7). This is presumably because the underlying lung substrate in patients with emphysema is more easily injured during surgery and takes longer to heal.

The role of emphysema as a risk factor for prolonged air leak has been inferred from numerous surgical case series which reliably demonstrate that patients noted pre-operatively to have emphysema will have a higher incidence of prolonged air leak. However, a major weakness of these studies, is that they are heterogenous in their definition of prolonged air leak, patient population (eg age, definition of impaired lung function), type of operation performed (eg video assisted vs open, chemical vs mechanical pleurodesis, type/extent of resection) and methods used to prevent air leak (eg use of pleural tenting), which limits the ability to compare between individual studies. In addition, several studies analyzing the specific risk factors for developing this complication have consistently shown that low FEV1 or FEV1/FVC will increase the risk of developing prolonged air leak after either pulmonary resection or lung volume reduction surgery (see below for details).

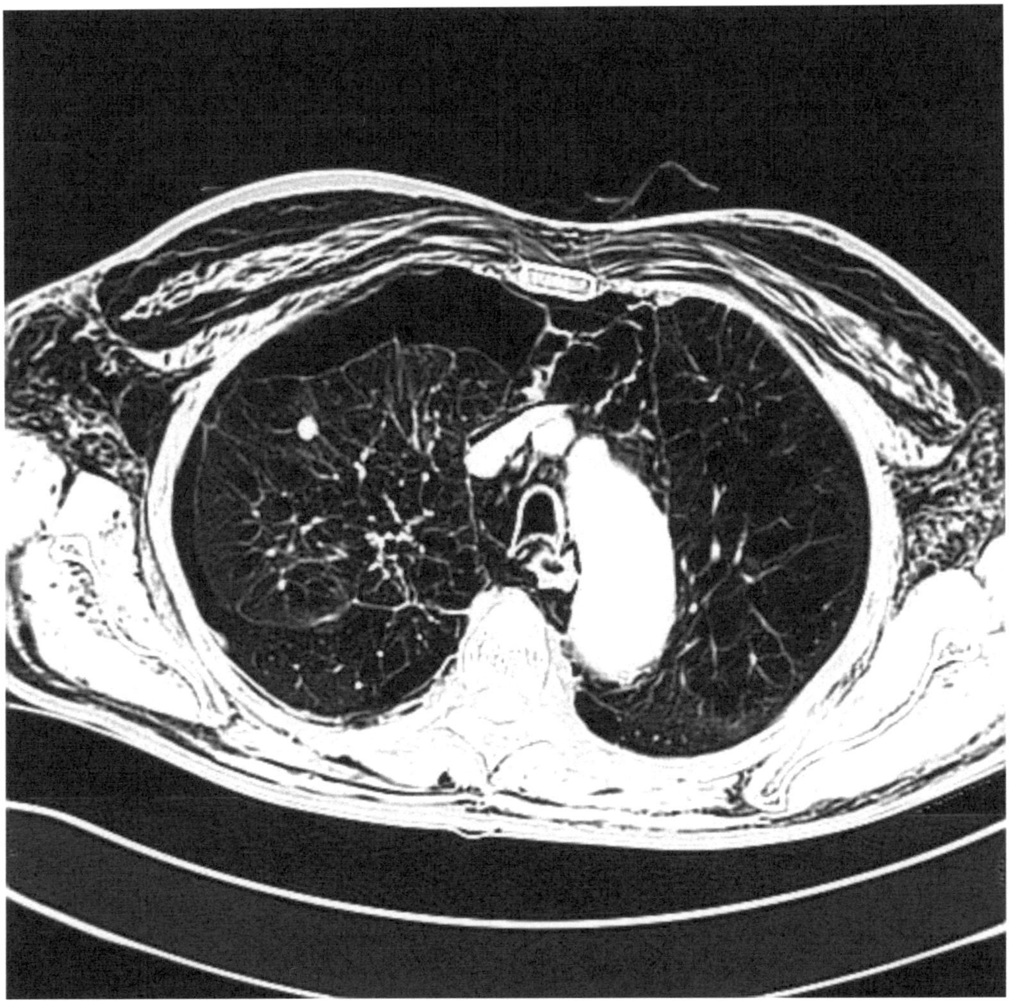

Fig. 1. Severe subcutaneous emphysema in a patient with underlying emphysema with prolonged air-leak.

For surgical pleurodesis, several authors have described their experience in performing this operation on both primary spontaneous pneumothorax and secondary spontaneous pneumothorax (which mainly consist of patients with underlying emphysema). The reported incidence of prolonged air leak in patients with primary spontaneous pneumothorax undergoing surgical pleurodesis has been reported to range from 0-3.8%, while it has been reported to range from 7.1-29.1% for patients with secondary spontaneous pneumothorax. A similar trend is also demonstrable in patients undergoing pulmonary resection for carcinoma of the lung, with an incidence of prolonged air leak of 4.2-18.2% in patients without underlying emphysema, compared to 5.4-44% in patients with underlying emphysema.

Author	Patient population	Type of pleurodesis	Definition of prolonged air leak (PAL)	Incidence of PAL in primary spontaneous pneumothorax	Incidence of PAL in secondary spontaneous pneumothorax
Hatz et al. (22)	95 patients with primary spontaneous pneumothorax requiring surgery 14 patients with secondary spotaneous pneumothorax requiring surgery (5 COPD patients)	VATS, excision of blebs, pleurectomy or talc powder (mechanical or chemical pleurodesis)	>2 days	2.1%	7.1%
Mouroux et al. (23)	75 patients with primary spontaneous pneumothorax requiring surgery 22 patients with secondary spontaneous pneumothorax requiring surgery (13 COPD patients)	VATS, excision of blebs, pleural abrasion or pleurectomy (mechanical pleurodesis)	>7 days	0 (excluded 1 patient who required conversion to open thoracotomy)	16.7% (excluded 4 patients who required conversion to open thoracotomy)
Noppen et al. (24)	28 patients with 31 episodes primary spontaneous pneumothorax requiring surgery 20 patients with 23 episodes of secondary spontaneous pneumothorax requiring surgery (6 COPD patients)	VATS, bleb ablation by electrocautery, talc powder (chemical pleurodesis)	>24 hours	0	26%
Passlick et al. (25)	65 patients with primary spontaneous pneumothorax requiring surgery 34 patients with secondary spontaneous pneumothorax requiring surgery (24 COPD patients)	VATS, excision of blebs, pleural abrasion ± pleurectomy (mechanical pleurodesis)	>7 days	1.7% (excluded 6 patients who required conversion to open thoracotomy)	16.6% (excluded 10 patients who required conversion to open thoracotomy)
Shaikhreza et al. (26)	480 patients with 550 episodes of primary spontaneous pneumothorax requiring surgery 89 patients with 94 episodes of secondary spontaneous pneumothorax requiring surgery (all patients with COPD)	VATS, excision of blebs, pleural abrasion, pleurectomy or talc powder (mechanical or chemical pleurodesis)	>5 days	3.8%	14.9%

Author	Patient population	Type of pleurodesis	Definition of prolonged air leak (PAL)	Incidence of PAL in primary spontaneous pneumothorax	Incidence of PAL in secondary spontaneous pneumothorax
Tanaka et al. (27)	130 patients with 100 episodes of primary spontaneous pneumothorax requiring surgery 67 patients with 24 episodes of secondary spontaneous pneumothorax requiring surgery (22 COPD patients)	Open thoracotomy, excision of blebs, pleural abrasion	>5 days	3%	29.1%

Table 1. Studies comparing the incidence of prolonged air leak in patients with primary versus secondary spontaneous pneumothorax undergoing surgical pleurodesis.

Author	Patient population	Type of pulmonary resection	Definition of prolonged air leak (PAL)	Incidence of PAL in patients without COPD	Incidence of PAL in patients with COPD
Lee et al. (28)	133 patients with FEV1 >80% predicted 104 patients with FEV1<80% predicted	Pneumonectomy (9.8% vs 10.6%), bilobectomy (4.5% vs 6.7%), lobectomy (84.2% vs 81.7%), wedge resection (1.5% vs 1.0%)	Not defined	6.7% (excludes pneumonectomy patients)	5.4% (excludes pneumonectomy patients)
Santambrogio et al. (29)	45 patients with FEV1 >80% predicted 43 patients with FEV1 <80% predicted	Upper lobectomy (64.4% vs 58.1%), other lobectomy (35.6% vs 41.9%)	>7 days	13.3%	16.2%
Sekine et al. (30)	166 patients with FEV1 >70% predicted & FEV1/FVC>70% 78 patients with FEV1 <70% predicted & FEV/FVC<70%	Pneumonectomy (13.9% vs 18%), bilobectomy (13.9% vs 19.2%), lobectomy (68.7% vs 58.8%), segmentectomy and wedge resection (2.4% vs 3.9%)	>10 days	4.2% (excludes pneumonectomy patients)	18.8% (excludes pneumonectomy patients)
Subotic et al. (31)	47 patients with FEV1/FVC >70% 35 patient with FEV1/FVC<70%	Pneumonectomy (53.2% vs 28.6%), upper lobectomy (23.4% vs 34.3%), other lobectomy (23.4% vs 37.1%)	Not defined	18.2% (excludes pneumonectomy patients)	44% (excludes pneumonectomy patients)

Table 2. Studies comparing the incidence of prolonged air leak in patients with COPD versus those without COPD undergoing pulmonary resection.

Author	Patient population	Type of lung volume reduction surgery	Type of intra-operative adjuncts used	Definition of prolonged air leak (PAL)	Incidence of PAL
Ciccone et al. (32)	250 patients, mean pre-op FEV1 26% of predicted	Bilateral LVRS via median sternotomy	Pleural tenting	>7 days	45.2%
DeCamp et al. (12)	580 patients, mean pre-op FEV1 26.8% of predicted	Bilateral VATS (30%) Bilateral LVRS via median sternotomy (70%)	Variety of methods (not standardized) including buttressing, sealants, tenting and pleurodesis	>7 days	45%
Ledrer et al. (33)	23 patients, mean pre-op FEV1 25% of predicted	Bilateral VATS (61%) Bilateral LVRS via median sternotomy (39%)	Buttressed staple lines	>7 days	39%

Table 3. Studies reporting the incidence of prolonged air leak in patients undergoing lung volume reduction surgery.

For lung volume reduction surgery, the incidence of prolonged air leak is much higher, ranging from 39-45.2%. This is expected, as the operation is conducted on both lungs, and usually on patients with more advanced underlying lung disease.

This review will discuss the pathogenesis, risk factors, intra-operative and post-operative management strategies for prolonged air leak in patients with emphysema based on current available literature. In addition, we propose an algorithm for the management of prolonged air leak in this group of patients based on this discussion, and also define specific criteria for surgical intervention for prolonged air leak that we follow at our institution. Several recent reviews have previously discussed the problem of prolonged air leaks, but do not focus specifically on patients with emphysema(3, 4) or neglect to discuss the utility of surgical intervention in greater detail(2, 34) which we believe plays an important role for this challenging clinical problem, particularly in the small number (but no less important) of patients who are refractory to all other forms of therapy.

2. Pathogenesis and factors influencing incidence of prolonged air leak in patients with emphysema

Some degree of post-operative air leak is generally unavoidable in operations involving pulmonary resection or mobilization, usually reflective of an alveolo-pleural fistula arising from exposed alveoli, whereas more severe leaks suggest fistulas arising from larger, more proximal bronchi(5, 7). The duration of the leak is related to the severity of the air leak as well as the time taken for the exposed parenchyma to heal, which occurs via an inflammatory reaction that results in granulation tissue formation and fibrin deposition(7). Moreover, this process is widely accepted to be facilitated by re-expansion of the lung to allow contact between the lung and parietal pleura.

Thus, it would follow that factors that would increase the risk of prolonged air leak include impaired wound healing (older age, more severe underlying emphysema), greater intra-operative surgical trauma (re-operations, extensive adhesions) and incomplete lung expansion post-operatively. This has been confirmed by a number of studies on patients undergoing pulmonary resection which have looked at specific factors that influence the incidence of prolonged air leak, summarized below.

Though no study looked specifically at risk factors for prolonged air leak in patients with emphysema undergoing pulmonary resection, DeCamp and colleagues(12) analyzed the data from the surgical arm of the National Emphysema Treatment Trial and found that the following factors increase the risk developing air leak after lung volume reduction surgery:

- Caucasian race (however, only 4.7% of trial participants were from minorities, so there may be an element of selection bias)
- Inhaled (but not oral) steroid use
- Poorer pulmonary function (lower FEV1 predicted or DLCO predicted)
- Upper lobe disease
- Pleural adhesions

Whether this can be extrapolated to patients with emphysema undergoing other forms of thoracic operations has not been demonstrated.

Author	Patient population	Definition of prolonged air leak	Incidence of prolonged air leak	Risk factors identified
Abolhoda et al. (11)	100 patients undergoing open upper lobectomy	>7 days	26%	- FEV1/FVC <50%
Brunelli et al. (16)	588 patients undergoing open lobectomy or bilobectomy	>7 days	15.6%	- low predicted post-operative FEV1 - pleural adhesions - upper lobectomy
Brunelli et al. (35)	658 patients undergoing open lobectomy	>5 days	13%	- age >65 - FEV1 <80% predicted - pleural adhesions - BMI < 25.5
Cerfolio et al. (36)	669 patients undergoing lobectomy, segmentectomy or wedge resection	>4 days	8%	- male gender - FEV1 <79% predicted - steroid use - lobectomy as opposed to lesser resection
Isowa et al. (37)	138 patients undergoing open lobectomy or segmentectomy	>10 days	18.1%	- diabetes - low serum albumin

Author	Patient population	Definition of prolonged air leak	Incidence of prolonged air leak	Risk factors identified
Lee et al. (38)	580 patients undergoing open lobectomy or segmentectomy	>7 days	18.6%	- low FEV1 predicted - low DLCO2 predicted - pleural adhesions
Liberman et al. (14)	1393 patients undergoing open lobectomy or bilobectomy	>5 days	5.6%	- female gender - history of smoking - low FEV1 predicted
Rivera et al. (39)	24,113 patients undergoing open lobectomy, bilobectomy, segmentectomy, bulla resection or LVRS	>7 days	6.9%	- male gender - low BMI - high dyspnea score - pleural adhesions - upper lobe disease - type of resection (LVRS > bilobectomy > lobectomy / segmentectomy > bulla resection)
Stolz et al.(13)	134 patients undergoing open loebectomy	>7 days	9.7%	- FEV1 <70% and FEV/FVC<70%

Table 4. Studies analyzing risk factors for prolonged air leak in patients undergoing pulmonary resection.

Based on the above mentioned factors, methods geared to the prevention of prolonged air leaks aim to minimize intra-operative surgical trauma or ensure more complete lung expansion. These approaches can be broadly divided into intra-operative and post-operative strategies.

3. Intra-operative strategies for prevention of prolonged air leak

3.1 General

The thoracic surgeon should ensure that lung tissue is handled as carefully as possible during dissection and manipulation to ensure minimal trauma, particularly in patients with emphysema, where the underlying lung is fragile. Any obvious parenchymal tears that are identified during surgery should be repaired meticulously. In addition, the remaining lung should be completely mobilized and decortication should be performed if necessary to aid maximal re-expansion of remaining lung tissue after pulmonary resection.

3.2 Fissureless technique for lobectomy

Conventional lobectomy involves dissection of lung parenchyma within the fissures by sharp or blunt dissection for exposure of the pulmonary artery that may result in air leaks. The fissureless technique involves exposing the pulmonary artery without such dissection, only using staplers for division of lung parenchyma when it is required(40, 41).

Although the efficacy of this technique has not been studied in patients with emphysema specifically, two previous studies on a general population of patients undergoing pulmonary resection have shown that this technique significantly decreases the incidence of prolonged air leak. Gomez-Caro and associates(42) demonstrated in a randomized prospective study of 63 patients undergoing either lobectomy or bilobectomy, that the incidence of prolonged air leak (>5 days) in patients whom a fissureless technique was employed was 3.2%, compared to 21.8% for those in whom conventional dissection was performed. A more recent retrospective case control study by Ng et al.(43) looking at 93 patients undergoing right upper lobectomy only, revealed similar results, with patients in the fissureless technique group having an incidence of prolonged air leak (>7 days) of 7.6%, compared to 22.2% in patients in the conventional lobectomy group.

3.3 No cut plication (non-resectional) technique for lung volume reduction surgery

For lung volume reduction surgery, an alternative technique involving no cut plication has been described by various authors as having lower rates of prolonged air leak while having short to intermediate term improvement in pulmonary function comparable to conventional lung volume reduction surgery(44-47). With this alternative technique, lung tissue is folded up or pushed down onto itself before being stapled together instead of performing staple excision of lung tissue in traditional lung volume reduction surgery.

Swanson and colleagues reported that in their series of 50 procedures performed on 32 patients, the incidence of prolonged air leak (>7 days) was only 8.6%(44). In a series of 20 patients operated by Iwasaki and associates, they reported that no patient had an air leak beyond 5 days(45). The largest reported series of 66 patients at Tor Vergata University by Tacconi, Pompeo and Mineo, demonstrated an incidence of prolonged air leak (>7 days) of 18% in patients undergoing non-resectional lung volume reduction surgery under thoracic epidural anaesthesia, compared to 40% of patients in a control group undergoing conventional lung volume reduction surgery under general anaesthesia(48).

Moreover, Pompeo and colleagues at the Tor Vergata University also recently published a randomized control trial comparing 32 patients undergoing non-resectional lung volume reduction surgery with thoracic epidural anaesthesia against 31 patients undergoing conventional lung volume reduction surgery with general anaesthesia and found that the incidence of prolonged air leak in the former was 18.8% compared to 48.4% for the latter, while survival and improvement in post-operative pulmonary function were similar in both groups (49). The same group also compared the results of 41 patients undergoing non-resectional lung volume reduction surgery under thoracic epidural anaesthesia against 19 patients undergoing non-resectional lung volume reduction surgery under general anaesthesia, and found that the occurrence of prolonged air leak was similar between the two groups (12.1% vs 26.3%, p=0.26), which suggests that the type of lung volume reduction surgery rather than the type of anaesthesia was the main factor in determining risk of prolonged air leak(50).

The above published data indicate that this technique may potentially be superior to the traditional lung volume reduction surgical approach in terms of reducing morbidity from prolonged air leak. However, the long-term durability of pulmonary function improvement after plication is still not known, as the studies so far have only involved small numbers of patients and only limited follow-up, thus more research on this technique is required before its widespread adoption can be recommended.

3.4 Buttress material for staple lines

Another area of study in the intra-operative prevention of air leaks during thoracic surgery has been the use of buttress material for staple lines, which in theory would help reinforce the fragile staple lines and thus prevent air leak from these areas of weakness. A variety of buttress materials have been described for this purpose, both synthetic (eg polytetrafluoroethylene(51), polydioxanone(52)) and biological [bovine pericardial strips(53-56), bovine collagen(57), autologous parietal pleura(58)]. However, only a few have been investigated in clinical practice, the most widely studied of which are bovine pericardial strips. Unfortunately, the cost of using these are high(57), and the few small studies that have been performed on a general population of patients undergoing pulmonary resection have not shown a clear benefit(53, 54). Several studies directed at emphysema patients specifically have been performed with more consistent results, but these are limited to those undergoing lung volume reduction surgery or bullectomy(55, 56, 58). On the other hand, an analysis of factors influencing post-operative air leak in patients undergoing lung volume reduction surgery in the National Emphsema Treatment Trial did not find that use of staple line buttressing (regardless of material) helpful in preventing or shortening duration of air leak(12).

In summary, current evidence suggest that the use of buttressing staple lines in patients with emphysema undergoing lung volume reduction surgery or bullectomy may be useful in reducing incidence of prolonged air leak, but its use in other operations, particularly pulmonary resection has not been demonstrated.

A table summarizing the results of the various studies mentioned above is presented below.

Author	Butress material	Patient population	Definition of prolonged air leak	Incidence of prolonged air leak	Time to chest tube removal (mean)	Length of stay (mean)
Miller et al.(53)	Bovine pericardial strips + stapler vs stapler alone	80 patients undergoing open lobectomy (65) or segmentectomy (15)	N/A	N/A	5.9 vs 6.3 days, p=0.62	8 vs 9 days, p=0.24
Venuta et al.(54)	Bovine pericardial strips + stapler vs stapler alone vs conventional cautery, clamp and ties	30 patients undergoing open lobectomy	>7 days	0% vs 20% vs 10%	N/A	4.4 vs 7.8 vs 7.2 days
Hazelrigg et al.(55)	Bovine pericardial strips + stapler vs stapler alone	123 patients with emphysema undergoing unilateral VATS LVRS	N/A	N/A	7.9 vs 10.4 days, p=0.04	8.6 vs 11.4 days, p=0.03
Stammberger et al.(56)	Bovine pericardial strips + staplers vs stapler alone	65 patients with emphysema undergoing bilateral VATS LVRS	Not defined	15.6% vs 21.2%	7.6 vs 9.7 days, p=0.045	12.7 vs 15.7 days, p=0.14

Author	Butress material	Patient population	Definition of prolonged air leak	Incidence of prolonged air leak	Time to chest tube removal (mean)	Length of stay (mean)
Baysungur et al.(58)	Autologous pleura + stapler vs stapler alone	22 patients with emphysema undergoing open bullectomy	>7 days	0% vs 8.3%	2.7 vs 4.8 days, p=0.04	4.2 vs 5.9 days, p=0.09
Fischel et al.(57)	Bovine pericardial strips + staples vs Bovine collagen + staples	56 patients with emphysema undergoing bilateral VATS LVRS	>7 days	35.7% vs 44.6%	8.6 vs 10.4 days	N/A

Table 5. Studies comparing the utility of buttressing staple lines in preventing prolonged air leak.

3.5 Pulmonary sealants

Pulmonary sealants have been the focus of a large amount of research in the area of intra-operative prevention air leaks, with over a dozen studies on various types of sealants including fibrin glue(59-62), PEG-based sealants(63-70) and coated collagen patches(71-73). However, as with studies on other strategies, these papers have generally not focused on patients with emphysema, and individually these studies each have small cohort sizes with very mixed patient populations as well as varying methods for reporting efficacy.

Moreover, the overall results of these studies so far have found no clear advantage in their routine use on all patients(74). Thus, the use of sealants should best be reserved for patients at highest risk for developing post-operative prolonged air leak(35, 38), especially since rare complications, particularly empyema(63, 67, 75) may arise from the use of pulmonary sealants. Indeed, the studies which have focused on patients with emphysema have more consistently shown a significant reduction in the incidence of post-operative prolonged air leak and length of stay(62, 73).

Author	Surgical sealant	Patient population	Definition of prolonged air leak	Incidence of prolonged air leak	Time to chest tube removal (mean)	Length of stay (mean)
Fleisher et al.(59)	Fibrin glue vs none	28 patients undergoing open lobectomy	>7 days	14.3% vs 7.1%	6.0 vs 5.9 days, p=0.95	9.8 vs 11.5 days, p=0.21
Wong et al.(60)	Fibrin glue vs none	66 patients undergoing open lobectomy, segmentectomy or decortication	N/A	N/A	6 vs 6 days, p=0.8 (median)	8 vs 9 days, p=0.57 (median)
Fabian et al.(61)	Fibrin glue vs none	100 patients undergoing open bilobectomy, lobectomy, segmentectomy or wedge resection	>7 days	2% vs 16%, p=0.015	3.5 vs 5.0 days, p=0.02	4.6 vs 4.9 days, p=0.318

Author	Surgical sealant	Patient population	Definition of prolonged air leak	Incidence of prolonged air leak	Time to chest tube removal (mean)	Length of stay (mean)
Porte et al.(63)	PEG based sealant vs none	124 patients undergoing open bilobectomy or lobectomy	>6 days	13% vs 22%, p=not significant	N/A	9.2 vs 8.6 days, p=not significant
Wain et al.(64)	PEG based sealant vs none	172 patients undergoing open bilobectomy, lobectomy, segmentectomy or wedge resection	>7 days	2.5% vs 7%	4.5 vs 5.2 days, p=0.41	7.4 vs 10.1 days, p=0.78
Allen et al.(65)	PEG based sealant vs none	161 patients undergoing open bilobectomy, lobectomy, segmentectomy, wedge resection, decortications or LVRS	>7 days	14% vs 12%, p=0.813	6.8 vs 6.2 days, p=0.679 (median)	6 vs 7 days, p=0.04 (median)
De Leyn et al.(66)	PEG based sealant vs none	121 patients undergoing open lobectomy or segmentectomy	N/A	N/A	3.90 vs 3.92 days, p=0.559 (median)	13 vs 12 days, p=0.292 (median)
Macchiarini et al.(67)	PEG based sealant vs none	24 patients undergoing open bilobectomy, lobectomy or wedge resection	N/A	N/A	6.1 vs 6.9 days, p=0.9	13 vs 14.4 days, p=0.4
Venuta et al.(68)	PEG based sealant vs none	50 patients undergoing lobectomy	>7 days	8% vs 20%	5.6 vs 10 days, p=0.03	8 vs 11.6 days, p=0.009
D'Andrilli et al.(69)	PEG based sealant vs none	203 patients undergoing open bilobectomy, lobectomy, segmentectomy or wedge resection	N/A	N/A	N/A	5.7 vs 6.2 days, p=0.18
Tan et al.(70)	PEG based sealant vs none	121 patients undergoing open bilobectomy, lobectomy or wedge resection	N/A	N/A	4 vs 3 days (median)	6 vs 7 days (median)
Lang et al.(71)	Coated collagen patch vs none	189 patients undergoing open lobectomy	Not defined	4.2% vs 3.2%	N/A	N/A
Anegg et al.(72)	Coated collagen patch vs none	173 patients undergoing open lobectomy or segmentectomy	>7 days	24% vs 32.46%, p=0.282	5.1 vs 6.3 days, p=0.022	6.2 to 7.7 days, p=0.01

Author	Surgical sealant	Patient population	Definition of prolonged air leak	Incidence of prolonged air leak	Time to chest tube removal (mean)	Length of stay (mean)
Rena et al.(73)	Coated collagen patch vs none	60 patients with COPD undergoing open lobectomy or segmentectomy	>7 days	3.3% vs 26.7%, p=0.029	3.53 vs 5.9 days, p=0.002	5.87 vs 7.5 days, p=0.01
Moser et al.(62)	Fibrin glue vs none	25 patients with emphysema undergoing bilateral VATS LVRS	>7 days	4.5% vs 31.8%, p=0.031	2.83 vs 5.88 days, p<0.001	N/A
Tansley et al.(76)	Bovine based surgical adhesive vs none	52 patients undergoing open lobectomy, segmentectomy or other resection	N/A	N/A	4 vs 5 days, p=0.012 (median)	6 vs 7 days, p=0.004 (median)
Belcher et al. (75)	Bovine based surgical adhesive vs fibrin glue	102 patients undergoing open bilobectomy, lobectomy, segmentectomy, or other resection	>7 days	18% vs 23%, p=0.627	5 vs 5 days, p=0.473	8 vs 7 days, p=0.382

Table 6. Studies comparing the utility of pulmonary sealants in preventing prolonged air leak.

3.6 Minimizing post-resectional spaces

Minimizing the potential space left behind after pulmonary resection allows for a more complete apposition of the lung surface with the parietal pleura to encourage the resolution of any post-operative air leak. Usually this can be accomplished with straightforward means such as the proper placement of chest tubes, division of the inferior pulmonary ligament and lysis of all adhesions at the conclusion of surgery or the use of adequate analgesia, chest physiotherapy or bronchoscopy to clear the airways of mucus and blood post-operatively to promote maximal re-expansion of the residual lung (7). In the event that the above mentioned methods are insufficient, several techniques have been described, including the creation of a pleural tent, creation of a pneumoperitoneum or deliberate diaphragmatic paralysis.

Again, interpretation of the results of studies on these methods to reduce post-resectional spaces is complicated by the heterogenous inclusion criteria and method of reporting outcomes in these studies. Furthermore, almost none have looked specifically at patients with emphysema, thus making it difficult to simply extrapolate the results of these studies to patients with emphysema.

Nonetheless, amongst the methods mentioned previously, pleural tenting has been the most widely studied technique for preventing prolonged air leak by minimizing post-resectional spaces. This involves stripping the parietal pleural over the apex, which is then resutured over the chest wall to produce an extrapleural space(7, 77). It has been used as a means for controlling the size of the potential space post-pulmonary resection in the upper thoracic cavity, and thus has been predominantly studied in patients undergoing upper lobectomy.

In a retrospective review on risk factors for prolonged post-operative air leak, Brunelli and associates(16) noted that patients with upper lobectomies who underwent a pleural tent had a significantly decreased duration of air leak compared to those who did not undergo a similar adjunctive procedure. Nevertheless, he later published a retrospective case matched analysis comparing patients with prolonged air leak after pulmonary resection and those without, which did not demonstrate that pleural tenting conferred any protective effect(9). DeCamp et al.(12) in reviewing the factors influencing air leak post-lung volume reduction surgery in patients from the National Emphysema Treatment Trial also did not find a significant decrease in incidence or duration of air leak in patients who underwent tenting compared to those who did not undergo tenting.

In addition, a number of randomized prospective studies have also been performed to assess its efficacy, and in general, the studies conducted on pleural tenting have shown an overall beneficial effect in terms of decreasing incidence of air leak, time to chest tube removal and length of stay. However, this procedure adds to operative time and may cause bleeding(35) though these were not shown to be significantly increased compared to controls in the studies below.

The table below summarizes the results of the randomized prospective studies performed to evaluate this technique.

Author	Patient population	Definition of prolonged air leak	Incidence of prolonged air leak	Time to chest tube removal (mean)	Length of stay (mean)
Brunelli et al.(77)	200 patients undergoing open upper lobectomy or bilobectomy (100 with tenting vs 100 without)	>7 days	14% vs 32% p=0.003	7 vs 11.2 days, p<0.0001	8.2 vs 11.6 days, p<0.0001
Allama et al.(78)	48 patients undergoing open upper lobectomy (23 with tenting vs 25 without)	>5 days	9% vs 40%, p=0.02	4.6 vs 5.6 days, p=0.11	4.96 vs 5.7 days, p=0.05
Okur et al.(79)	40 patients undergoing open upper lobectomy or bilobectomy (20 with tenting vs 20 without)	>5 days	0 vs 30%	4.3 vs 7.4 days, p<0.0001	7.6 vs 9.35 days, p=0.024

Table 7. Studies comparing the utility of pleural tenting in preventing prolonged air leak.

Conversely, the creation a pneumoperitoneum has been utilized to minimize the post-resectional space in the lower thoracic cavity. This has been described as both an intra-operative adjunct to prevent prolonged air leak(80) as well as a post-operative technique(81-83) to treat it. It can be accomplished through instillation of air into the peritoneal cavity by a variety of means, including under direct vision through a transdiaphragmatic opening made in the diaphragm during surgery(80), via insertion of a peritoneal dialysis catheter under local anesthesia(81), or with the aid of a Veres needle under local anesthesia(82, 83) .

A small randomized prospective trial by Cerfolio and colleagues(80) studied 16 patients undergoing right middle and lower bilobectomy, dividing them into a group who underwent intra-operative pneumoperitoneum creation and a group who did not undergo this procedure. 0/8 patients with an intra-operative pneumoperitoneum had air leak by POD3, compared to 4/8 patients who did not have an intra-operative pneumoperitoneum ($p<0.001$). Moreover, patients in the former group had a median hospitalization stay of 4 days compared to 6 days for patients in the latter group ($p<0.001$). Thus, this is an interesting technique, but conclusions on its efficacy are difficult to draw based on the limited data available. The results of post-operative pneumoperitoneum creation will be discussed later in the section on post-operative strategies for management of prolonged air leak.

Deliberate diaphragmatic paralysis is an alternative method used to decrease the potential space in the lower thoracic cavity to allow for more rapid resolution of air leak. Several means are available to achieve this, including infiltration of the phrenic nerve with local anesthetic, phrenic nerve crush or sectioning. The main drawback of diaphragmatic paralysis is the compromise in ventilatory function and cough mechanism. Thus, the use of para-phrenic local anesthetic has the advantage over phrenic nerve crush or sectioning, in that it only resulting in temporary paralysis, so that diaphragmatic function may recover after the effect of the local anesthetic wears off. A recent case report by Clavero and associates(84) explains how an epidural catheter can be placed in close proximity of the phrenic nerve through video-assisted thoracoscopic surgery or thoracotomy, so that the managing physician can dictate the exact duration of diaphragmatic paralysis required to resolve the air leak before reversing the effect of the local anesthetic infusion. However, no large studies specifically describing the use of diaphragmatic paralysis for preventing prolonged air leaks are available.

4. Post-operative strategies for management of prolonged air leak

4.1 Bronchoscopy and endobronchial techniques

Bronchoscopy plays an important role in the post-operative management of prolonged air leak. It can be used to clear the airways of mucus and blood to aid maximal re-expansion of the lung to promote resolution of air leaks. Furthermore, it should be performed in all patients with persistent air leak to exclude stump dehiscence, as its presence will often necessitate surgery to treat the problem. Should surgery be contraindicated for whatever reason, a large number of endobronchial approaches have been studied as an alternative therapeutic option for bronchopleural fistulas, including the use of glue(85, 86), polidocanol(87), tetracycline(88), coils(89), surgicel(90), gelfoam(91), tracheobronchial stents(92), atrial septal defect closure devices(93) and even lasers(94). Unfortunately, experience with these techniques have been limited to mostly case reports and case series, with no controlled studies comparing the different methods or comparing them against surgical therapy. A recent systematic review of several of the larger case series by West et al. (95) showed that among 85 patients with post-pneumonectomy bronchopleural fistulas, endobronchial therapy (40 fibrin glue, 15 cyanoacrylate glue, 19 polidocanol, 6 lasers, 5 stents) succeeded in treating only 30% of them. Overall mortality was 40%, with many patients requiring multiple bronchoscopic procedures or additional surgical drainage.

In addition, the placement of endobronchial valves is a new technique that has emerged recently for the treatment of persistent air leak in patients with underlying lung disease such as emphysema that are not candidates for more extensive procedures such as surgery(96, 97). Endobronchial one-wave valves inserted via bronchoscopy were initially developed as an investigational technique to treat emphysema by promoting atelectasis of emphysematous lungs distal to the valve, which would allow air to exit via the valve but not re-enter. They have now been used in selected patients with persistent air leaks, in hope that they accelerate closure of the leak by minimizing flow of air through the leak(98).

The procedure can be performed either under sedation or general anesthesia, using either a flexible or rigid bronchoscope. A balloon tipped catheter is used to provide selective bronchial occlusion to determine the segmental or subsegmental airway that results in the greatest decrease in air leak. The endobronchial valve is then inserted in these airways (98, 99). The results of the two largest series on endobronchial valve placement are summarized below, and the overall conclusion is it is a promising mode of therapy particularly for patients with no other therapeutic options.

Author	Patient population	Duration of air leak prior to valve placement (median)	Number of patients with improvement	Duration of chest tube drainage after valve placement (median)	Duration of hospitalization after valve placement (median)	Complications
Travaline et al.(98)	40 patients with underlying lung disease (30% COPD) that had persistent air leaks (17.5% post-operative)	20 days	37 (92.5%)	7.5 days	11 days	6 (valve expectoration, malpositioning of the valve requiring redeployment, pneumonia, oxygen desaturation and MRSA colonization)
Gillespie et al.(99)	7 patients with underlying lung disease (71% COPD) that had persistent air leaks (71% post-operative)	28 days	7 (100%)	16 days	3 days	Nil

Table 8. Studies reporting the efficacy of endobronchial valve placement in the treatment of prolonged air leak.

4.2 Bedside pleurodesis

Instillation of a sclerosing agent into the pleural space elicits an inflammatory reaction in the pleura that allows for the obliteration of the pleural space and resolution of an air leak. A variety of agents have been described for this purpose, including silver nitrate(100), quinacrine(101), minocycline(102), tetracycline(103), doxycycline(104), erythromycin(105), bleomycin(106), iodopovidone(107), talc powder(14) and autologous blood(108-111). Be that as it may, contemporary literature has mainly focused on autologous blood for treatment of persistent post-operative air leaks, so the utility of the other agents for this clinical context are not as well known. Also, these studies were not limited to patients with emphysema, so their results may not be directly applicable for these patients with persistent post-operative air leaks. However, based on available published data, bedside pleurodesis is a reasonably efficacious modality of treatment with few adverse effects, so it is often used as first line therapy for patients with prolonged air leak, even in our own institution.

Several small observational studies have demonstrated the efficacy and safety of autologous blood in treating post-operative prolonged air leak(108-110). In these studies, patients with prolonged air leak (>5-10 days) after undergoing a variety of operations (lobectomy, wedge resection, bullectomy, lung volume reduction or decortication) were treated with 1-2 injections of autologous blood pleurodesis with resolution of air leak in all patients within 48 hours of therapy. No major complications occurred except for fever, pneumonia or prolonged pleural effusion in a minority of patients.

In addition, Shackcloth et al.(111) performed a randomized prospective study on 20 post-lobectomy patients with prolonged air leak (>5 days) to evaluate autologous blood pleurodesis compared to controls. They showed that there was a statistically significant ($p<0.001$) reduction in median time to chest tube removal (6.5 vs 12 days) and hospital discharge (8 vs 13.5 days) with autologous blood pleurodesis. One patient in the pleurodesis arm however developed an empyema.

As for the other forms of chemical pleurodesis, Liberman and associates(14) reported their experience with 41 patients who underwent chemical pleurodesis (30 talc, 7 doxycycline, 1 doxycycline+talc, 1 bleomycin, 1 bleomycin+talc) for prolonged air leak (>5 days) after undergoing lobectomy or bilobectomy. Sclerosis was successful in 40 patients (97.6%), with the remaining one patient having to undergo a pectoralis major flap for persistent air leak despite talc pleurodesis. Also, one patient developed empyema after talc pleurodesis.

As indicated above, complications of bedside pleurodesis include mainly consist of fever, pain and empyema. In addition, the most feared complication of talc pleurodesis is a systemic inflammatory response to talc that can result in acute respiratory distress syndrome(112, 113) particularly if the talc particle size is small(114). However, it has previously been found to be not associated with increased mortality in a meta-analysis of patients with malignant pleural effusion undergoing talc pleurodesis(115).

4.3 Post-operative creation of pneumoperitoneum

As mentioned previously, the creation of a pneumoperitoneum has been described as both an intra-operative as well as a post-operative method of controlling prolonged air leaks. This involves the instillation of air into the peritoneal cavity via insertion of a peritoneal dialysis catheter under local anesthesia(81), or with the aid of a Veres needle under local anesthesia(82, 83). The creation of a pneumoperitoneum is often combined with a form of pleural sclerosis, such as talc(81, 82) or autologous blood(83), to aid the resolution of air leak. Several potential disadvantages of this technique include the risk of insertion of peritoneal dialysis catheter / Veres needle (eg bleeding, injury to intra-abdominal viscera) and possible respiratory compromise from the creation of the pneumoperitoneum.

Not many studies have been performed to evaluate this modality of therapy, except for a few isolated case reports, so the technique has shown promise in treatment of some patients but has not been evaluated on a large scale basis. Handy and associates(81) reported the successful use of this technique to resolve a persistent air leak of more than 3 weeks duration in a patient with emphysema who underwent lung volume reduction surgery. De Giacomo and colleagues(82) described the use of post-operative pneumoperitoneum to manage persistent air leak (>5 days) in 14 patients who underwent pulmonary resection for lung cancer, with resolution of the air leak occurring within 4-12 (mean 8) days after the procedure. The most recent paper assessing this technique by Korasidis et al.(83) demonstrated that combined post-operative pneumoperitoneum and autologous blood patch was able to control prolonged air leak (>3 days) present in 39 patients who underwent pulmonary resection for lung cancer within 144 hours of therapy. No major complications with the technique were reported by any of the above studies.

4.4 Optimal chest tube management and outpatient chest tube management

Appropriate chest tube management has also been shown to influence the duration of post-operative air leak. With respect to chest tube suction, it may be viewed in one of two ways. Firstly, chest tube suction may promote pleural apposition to decrease duration of air leaks, or alternatively, suction may cause tension on suture lines to prolong air leaks. The experience in lung volume reduction surgery had previously demonstrated that duration of prolonged air leak was decreased by avoiding routine chest tube suction in these patients(116).

This was subsequently investigated in several randomized prospective studies to see if this also held true in patients undergoing other forms of thoracic operations. For patients undergoing apical pleurectomy following primary spontaneous pneumothorax, Ayed demonstrated that converting to water seal (no suction) after a period of initial active suction significantly decreased the risk of prolonged air leak and duration of chest tube drainage compared to active suction throughout(117). A similar benefit of converting to water seal after a period of initial active suction for patients undergoing pulmonary resection (lobectomy, segmentectomy or wedge resections) was demonstrated by two separate groups(118, 119). However, a comparable study by Brunelli and associates(120) showed that water seal had no advantage over active suction when limited to a population of patients undergoing lobectomy. A follow-up study demonstrated that in patients undergoing lobectomy, alternate suction (at night) and water seal (during the day) was better than water seal alone(121).

A different approach was evaluated by Alphonso and colleagues, who studied a mixed cohort of patients undergoing a variety of operations (VATS as well as open lobectomy, wedge resections, lung biopsies or pneumothorax operations) and found that adopting water seal immediately after surgery showed no difference in air leak duration compared to active suction(122).

Whether these approaches are applicable to patients with underlying emphysema undergoing pulmonary resection or pleurodesis has yet to be conclusively demonstrated, but a strategy of minimizing duration of chest tube suction or alternating it with water seal would be prudent based on evidence available so far. In addition, it should be noted that patients on water seal, particularly those with large air leaks, should be monitored for evidence of increasing subcutaneous emphysema or enlarging pneumothorax, as these patients will need to be placed back on active suction to prevent clinical deterioration(118).

Author	Patient population	Chest tube management	Definition of prolonged air leak	Incidence of prolonged air leak	Time to chest tube removal (mean)
Ayed(117)	100 patients undergoing VATS pleurodesis for primary spontaneous pneumothorax	Initial chest tube suction, then water seal vs active suction throughout	>5 days	2% vs 14% (p=0.03)	2.7 vs 3.8 days (p=0.004)
Cerfolio et al.(118)	33 patients undergoing bilobectomy, lobectomy, segmentectomy or wedge resection	Initial chest tube suction, then water seal vs active suction throughout	NA	NA	NA
Marshall et al.(119)	68 patients undergoing lobectomy, segmentectomy or wedge resection	Initial chest tube suction, then water seal vs active suction throughout	NA	NA	3.33 vs 5.47 days (p=0.06)
Brunelli et al.(120)	145 patients undergoing bilobectomy or lobectomy	Initial chest tube suction, then water seal vs active suction throughout	>7 days	27.8% vs 30.1% (p=0.8)	11.5 vs 10.3 (p=0.2)
Brunelli et al.(121)	94 patients undergoing bilobectomy or lobectomy	Initial chest tube suction, then water seal vs alternating suction (at night) and water seal (during the day)	>7 days	19% vs 4% (p=0.02)	8.6 vs 5.2 days (p=0.002)
Alphonso et al.(122)	239 patients undergoing lobectomy, segmentectomy, wedge resection or pneumothorax operations	Immediate water seal vs active suction throughout	>6 days	10.1% vs 7.8% (p=0.62)	NA

Table 9. Studies comparing the utility of chest tube management strategies in preventing prolonged air leak.

An alternative strategy to prolonged air leaks is the use of Heimlich valves or portable chest drainage systems to allow for early discharge of patients who are otherwise ready to be discharged from hospital apart from their prolonged air leak. Heimlich valves are one way valves originally used for the outpatient management of a pneumothorax, and two studies have shown that they can be successfully used to discharge select patients with prolonged air leak early with relatively few complications(123, 124). Portable chest tube drainage systems have an additional advantage over Heimlich valves in that they are able to handle fluid drainage in addition to air leak and can also be connected to active suction when required(125). In conclusion, outpatient chest tube management appears to be an acceptable approach that is fairly safe for managing most patients with prolonged air leak if they are reliable enough to handle their Heimlich valve or portable chest tube system on their own at home.

Author	Patient population	Type of outpatient chest tube management	Duration of outpatient chest tube management (mean)	Complications
McKenna et al.(124)	25 patients post-lung volume reduction surgery with prolonged air leak (> 5 days)	Heimlich valve	7.7 days	Nil
Ponn et al.(123)	45 patients post lobectomy, wedge resection or bullectomy with prolonged air leak (not defined)	Heimlich valve	7.5 days	1 pneumonia
Rieger et al.(125)	36 patients post-lobectomy, segmentectomy, wedge resection, pleurodesis, pericardial window, mediastinal dissection or esophagogastrectomy with prolonged air leak or excessive drainage	Portable chest tube system with suction	11.2 days	1 cellulitis, 1 localized empyema, 1 recurrence of pneumothorax

Table 10. Studies reporting the use of Heimlich valves or portable chest tube systems in the outpatient treatment of prolonged air leak.

As to which patients with prolonged air leak are suitable for discharge without suction, Cerfolio and colleagues(126) reported that they successfully discharged 199 post-pulmonary resection patients with a suctionless portable device safely without complications as long as there was no development of a new or enlarging pneumothorax or subcutaneous emphysema after converting the original chest tube suction to water seal. More importantly, most of these patients had their air leak resolve by the end of 2 weeks of outpatient chest tube therapy, and for the remaining 57 who still had air leak, the chest tube was safely removed if these patients were asymptomatic, had no increase in pneumothorax or new subcutaneous emphysema on the outpatient device. There were no complications except for the development of empyema in 3 of these 57 patients (5.7%), but these 3 patients were immunocompromised and were on chronic steroid therapy.

4.5 Re-operation

If all else fails, in cases of persistent air leak that is refractory to methods described above, re-operation can be considered to look for the source of air leak and perform therapeutic maneuvers. Often this can be accomplished with video assisted thoracoscopy, such as described by Suter and associates(127), who managed to identify the source of air leak thoracoscopically in 3 patients who had prolonged air leak after pulmonary resection. The air leaks were subsequently sealed with direct application of fibrin glue or pleurodesis with silver nitrate.

However, patients with massive, severe prolonged air leaks, particularly those with a concomitant large pleural space problem, usually require a more extensive operation such as a thoracoplasty or muscle flap transposition via an open thoracotomy. Thoracoplasty, the reduction of thoracic cavity by removal of ribs, is rarely done as it results in thoracic deformity, restriction in shoulder mobility and decreased respiratory function(7, 128). As such, muscular flap transpositions have become the preferred technique, and we have developed the combined latissimus dorsi-serratus anterior transposition flap for this purpose. We have previously described 5 patients who underwent this technique (two COPD patients with pneumothorax refractory to conservative management, one COPD patient with prolonged air leak post lung volume reduction surgery, two patients with bronchopleural fistula/empyemas), with resolution of air leak that allows the chest tubes to be removed within 5 days after surgery and no recurrence of air leak noted at 1 year follow-up(129).

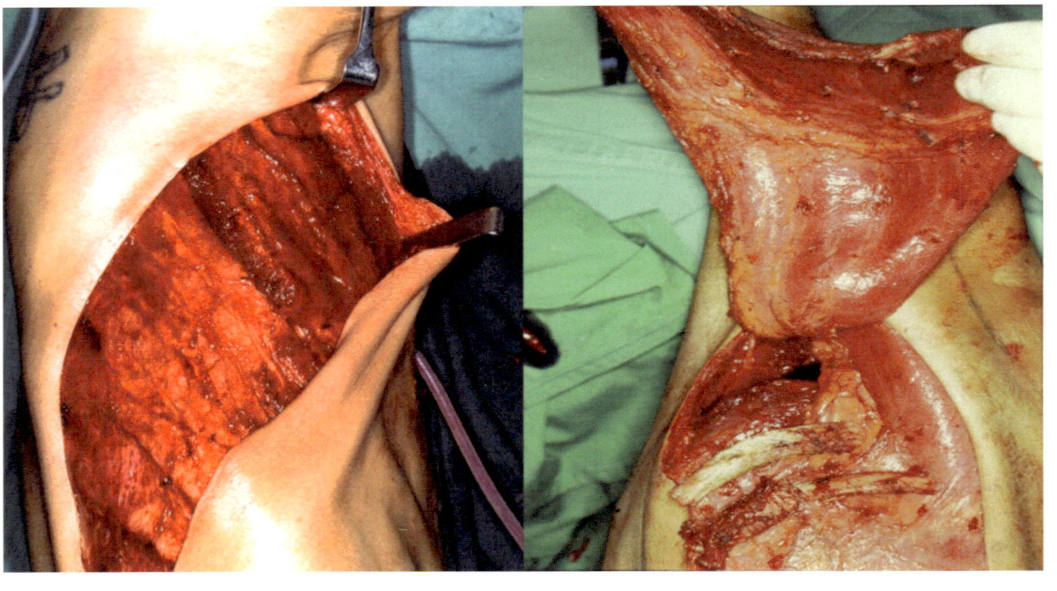

Fig. 2. (a) The latissimus dorsi and proximal slips of the serratus anterior are raised as pedicled flaps via a lazy S incision from mid-axillary line to the inferior limit of the latissimus dorsi. An axillary window is then created by resecting the 2nd and 3rd ribs superior to the serratus anterior.

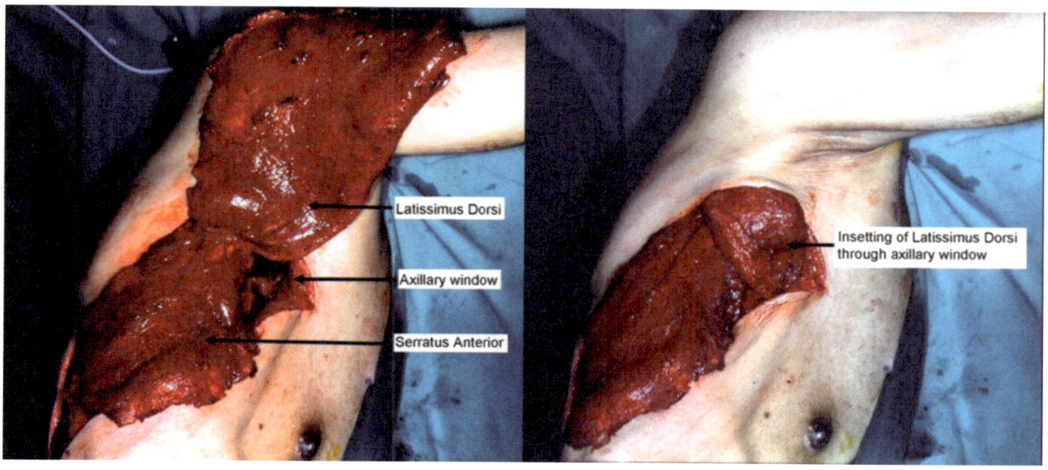

Fig. 2. (b) Latissimus dorsi and serratus anterior reflected to demonstrate the axillary window. The latissimus dorsi flap is then passed though the axillary window and laid over the lung to obliterate the pleural space and seal the air leak.

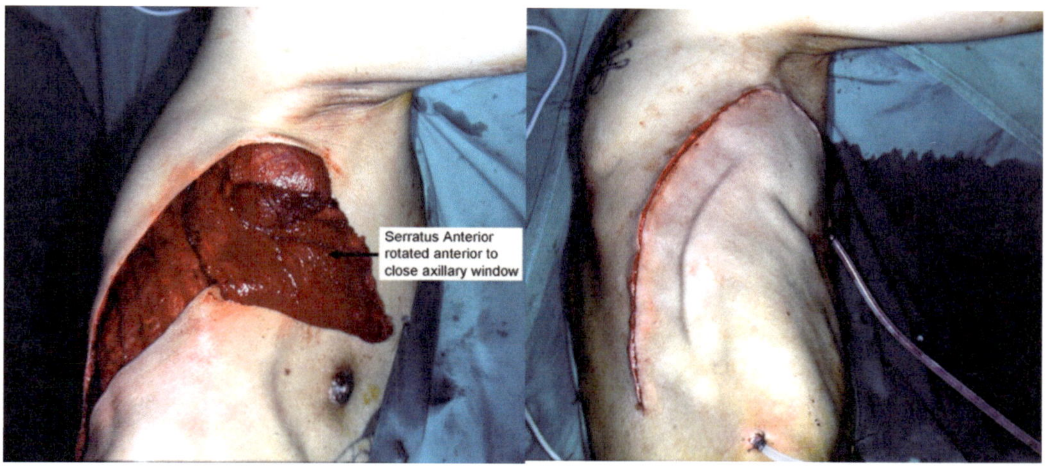

Fig. 2. (c) Serratus anterior flap is rotated anteriorly over the latissimus dorsi flap to close the axillary window. Primary closure of the incision was then performed.

At our institution, our indications for surgical air leak repair with flap reconstruction are (1) severe air leaks (high leak rate or continuous leak despite application of chest tube suction), (2) persistent air leak exceeding 4 weeks despite conservative management (or beyond 1 week for patients with underlying lung disease such as COPD), and (3) significant pleural dead space defined radiologically by absence of pleural-pleural contact despite maximal re-expansion efforts(16, 36, 130).

The operation is performed via a muscle sparing posterolateral thoracotomy with a lazy-S incision extending from the axilla to the lumbar region. Then, the latissimus dorsi and the serratus anterior muscle flaps are raised, with care taken to ensure that the serratus anterior flap is sufficient to cover the intended axillary window (usually by raising muscle slips from the 2nd to 4th ribs) but sparing the lower slips of muscle that insert into the scapula to avoid scapular winging. Creation of the axillary window involves resection of the second to fourth ribs centered over the mid-axillary line which allows good exposure of the underlying lung for surgical treatment (eg suture repair of parenchymal tears, decortication) and allows the latissimus dorsi to the passed through without compressing its vascular pedicle. The latissimus dorsi is loosely anchored over the lung and a chest tube is inserted after a final check for air leak. The axillary window is then closed with the serratus anterior muscle flap and the skin incision is closed over a subcutaneous drain.

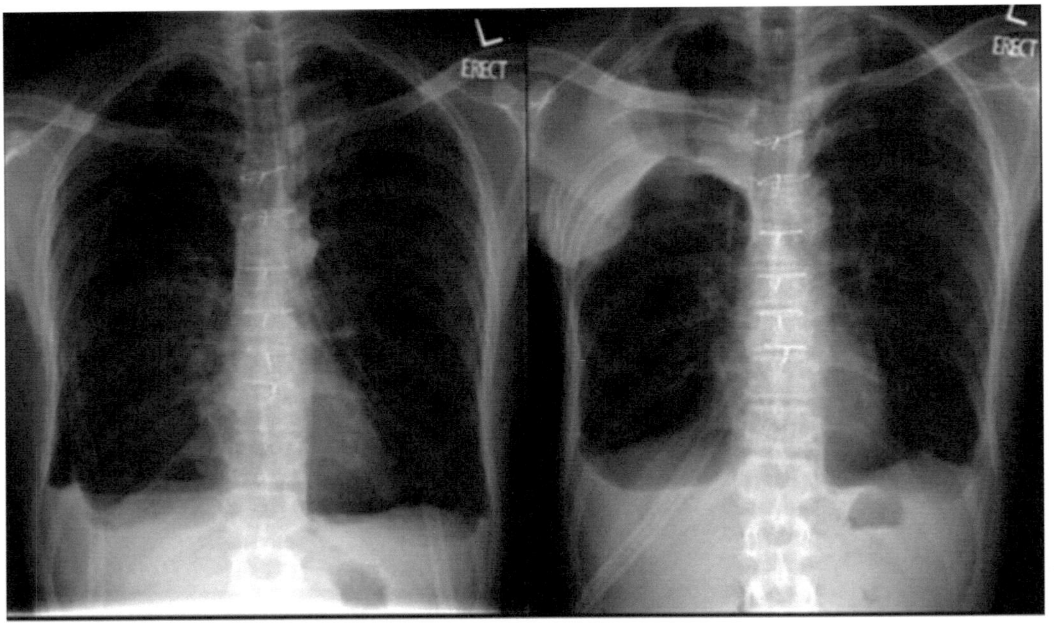

Fig. 3. Pre-operative chest x-ray (left) showing a large potential pleural space with resulting persistent air leak in this patient who had underwent bilateral lung volume reduction surgery, and post-operative chest x-ray (right) showing effective re-expansion of the right lung after the placement of the latissimus dorsi flap.

We believe our technique has several distinct advantages, as firstly it offers direct visualization for repair of diseased lung parenchyma via an open thoracotomy. Secondly, the latissimus dorsi flap provides a large, well vascularised surface for the lung to adhere to for healing. Moreover, the large mass of the muscle eliminates any pleural dead space and facilitates subsequent controlled re-expansion of the lung with time. Finally, the serratus anterior flap compartmentalizes the pleural cavity from the large subcutaneous space created by the latissimus dorsi harvest to prevent seroma formation or spread of infection between compartments. Minimal functional disability occurs after these muscle harvests, and scapular winging is prevented by sparing the lower slips of the serratus anterior muscle and the long thoracic nerve. This is in contrast to other methods for reducing pleural dead space which may only be sufficient to deal with a small volume of space (pleural tenting, pneumoperitoneum), or reduces the patient's functional lung reserve (phrenic nerve paralysis, thoracoplasty).

Other muscular flaps that have been described in contemporary literature to eliminate potential pleural spaces (though these have been traditionally ascribed for managing empyema spaces rather than persistent air leaks) include isolated pectoralis major (14, 131), latissimus dorsi (131, 132), serratus anterior (131), rectus abdominis(131, 133) and the trapezius flaps (131, 134). However, we have found in our own experience that these flaps either lack the reach or necessary bulk in order to properly treat the large pleural space problems that we have encountered. Thus, we feel that this combination muscle flap technique is an important and useful tool in the thoracic surgeon's armamentarium in dealing with recalcitrant post-operative air leaks in a variety of situations, particularly in patients with a background of impaired respiratory function such as severe emphysema.

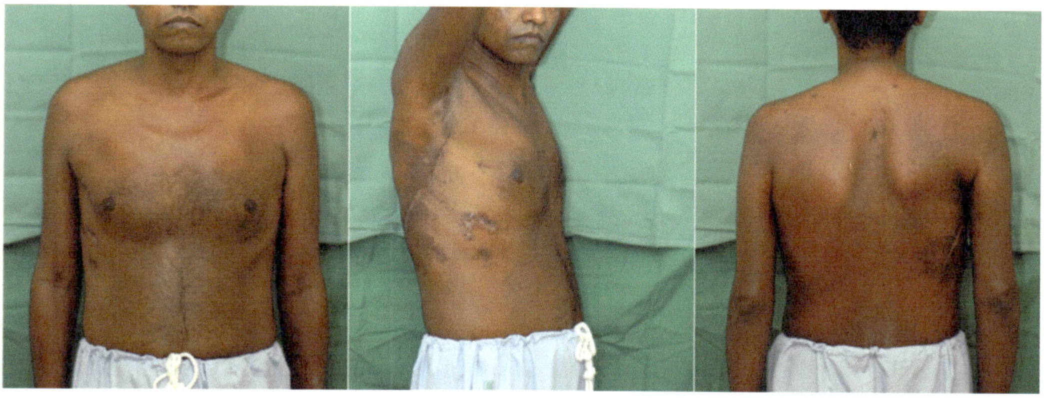

Fig. 4. Two months after the initial operation, this patient has good recovery of shoulder function.

5. Summary

In summary, prolonged air leak is a common problem for patients with emphysema undergoing thoracic surgery that is associated with significant morbidity. Clinicians involved in the surgical care of this group of patients should be aware of the various factors which can further increase the risk of this complication occurring and need to know the various measures that should be employed to prevent this problem, as well as the treatment options available should prolonged air leak occur even if preventive measures are taken. Based on the review of best available evidence as discussed previously, we propose a suggested algorithm for the management of prolonged air leaks in patients with emphysema with gradual progression of therapy similar to what has been proposed by others(2-4) but that also takes into account criteria for surgical intervention as we have mentioned earlier.

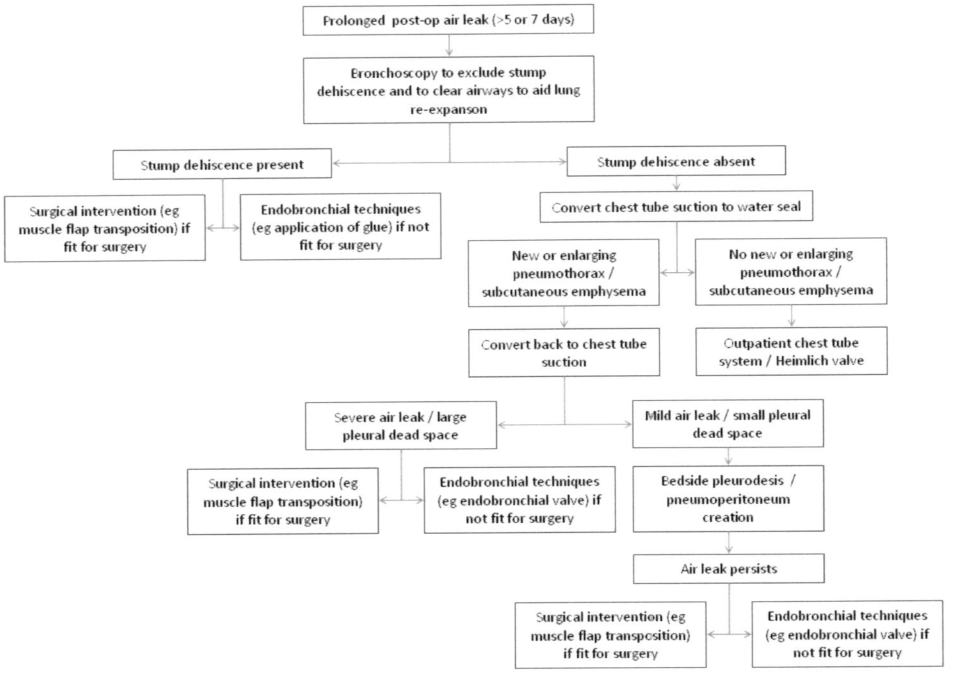

Fig. 5. Proposed algorithm for the management of prolonged air leaks in patients with emphysema.

6. References

[1] Haithcock BE, Feins RH. Complications of pulmonary resection. In: Shields TW, LoCicero J, Reed CE, Feins RH, editors. General Thoracic Surgery. 7th ed. Philadelphia: Lippincott Williams & Wilkins; 2009. p. 552-9.

[2] Shrager JB, DeCamp MM, Murthy SC. Intraoperative and postoperative management of air leaks in patients with emphysema. Thorac Surg Clin. 2009 May;19(2):223-31, ix.

[3] Singhal S, Ferraris VA, Bridges CR, Clough ER, Mitchell JD, Fernando HC, et al. Management of alveolar air leaks after pulmonary resection. Ann Thorac Surg. 2010 Apr;89(4):1327-35.

[4] Merritt RE, Singhal S, Shrager JB. Evidence-based suggestions for management of air leaks. Thorac Surg Clin. 2010 Aug;20(3):435-48.

[5] Burke SJ, Faber LP. Complications of pulmonary resection. In: Little AG, editor. Complications in Cardiothoracic Surgery: Avoidance and Treatment. 1st ed. New York: Futura; 2004. p. 67-91.

[6] Dexter EU, Kohman LJ. Perioperative care of patients undergoing thoracic surgery. In: Sellke FW, del Nido PJ, Swanson SJ, editors. Sabiston & Spencer Surgery of the Chest. 7th ed. Philadelphia: Saunders; 2004. p. 43-57.

[7] Deslauriers J, Mehran R. Handbook of Perioperative Care in General Thoracic Surgery. Philadelphia: Mosby; 2005.

[8] Okereke I, Murthy SC, Alster JM, Blackstone EH, Rice TW. Characterization and importance of air leak after lobectomy. Ann Thorac Surg. 2005 Apr;79(4):1167-73.

[9] Brunelli A, Xiume F, Al Refai M, Salati M, Marasco R, Sabbatini A. Air leaks after lobectomy increase the risk of empyema but not of cardiopulmonary complications: a case-matched analysis. Chest. 2006 Oct;130(4):1150-6.
[10] Varela G, Jimenez MF, Novoa N, Aranda JL. Estimating hospital costs attributable to prolonged air leak in pulmonary lobectomy. Eur J Cardiothorac Surg. 2005 Feb;27(2):329-33.
[11] Abolhoda A, Liu D, Brooks A, Burt M. Prolonged air leak following radical upper lobectomy: an analysis of incidence and possible risk factors. Chest. 1998 Jun;113(6):1507-10.
[12] DeCamp MM, Blackstone EH, Naunheim KS, Krasna MJ, Wood DE, Meli YM, et al. Patient and surgical factors influencing air leak after lung volume reduction surgery: lessons learned from the National Emphysema Treatment Trial. Ann Thorac Surg. 2006 Jul;82(1):197-206; discussion -7.
[13] Stolz AJ, Schutzner J, Lischke R, Simonek J, Pafko P. Predictors of prolonged air leak following pulmonary lobectomy. Eur J Cardiothorac Surg. 2005 Feb;27(2):334-6.
[14] Liberman M, Muzikansky A, Wright CD, Wain JC, Donahue DM, Allan JS, et al. Incidence and risk factors of persistent air leak after major pulmonary resection and use of chemical pleurodesis. Ann Thorac Surg. 2010 Mar;89(3):891-7; discussion 7-8.
[15] Irshad K, Feldman LS, Chu VF, Dorval JF, Baslaim G, Morin JE. Causes of increased length of hospitalization on a general thoracic surgery service: a prospective observational study. Can J Surg. 2002 Aug;45(4):264-8.
[16] Brunelli A, Monteverde M, Borri A, Salati M, Marasco RD, Fianchini A. Predictors of prolonged air leak after pulmonary lobectomy. Ann Thorac Surg. 2004 Apr;77(4):1205-10; discussion 10.
[17] Noppen M, De Keukeleire T. Pneumothorax. Respiration. 2008;76(2):121-7.
[18] Sahn SA, Heffner JE. Spontaneous pneumothorax. N Engl J Med. 2000 Mar 23;342(12):868-74.
[19] Rooney C, Sethi T. The epithelial cell and lung cancer: the link between chronic obstructive pulmonary disease and lung cancer. Respiration. 2011;81(2):89-104.
[20] Molina JR, Yang P, Cassivi SD, Schild SE, Adjei AA. Non-small cell lung cancer: epidemiology, risk factors, treatment, and survivorship. Mayo Clin Proc. 2008 May;83(5):584-94.
[21] Criner GJ, Cordova F, Sternberg AL, Martinez FJ. The NETT: Part II- Lessons Learned about Lung Volume Reduction Surgery. Am J Respir Crit Care Med. 2011 Jun 30.
[22] Hatz RA, Kaps MF, Meimarakis G, Loehe F, Muller C, Furst H. Long-term results after video-assisted thoracoscopic surgery for first-time and recurrent spontaneous pneumothorax. Ann Thorac Surg. 2000 Jul;70(1):253-7.
[23] Mouroux J, Elkaim D, Padovani B, Myx A, Perrin C, Rotomondo C, et al. Video-assisted thoracoscopic treatment of spontaneous pneumothorax: technique and results of one hundred cases. J Thorac Cardiovasc Surg. 1996 Aug;112(2):385-91.
[24] Noppen M, Meysman M, d'Haese J, Monsieur I, Verhaeghe W, Schlesser M, et al. Comparison of video-assisted thoracoscopic talcage for recurrent primary versus persistent secondary spontaneous pneumothorax. Eur Respir J. 1997 Feb;10(2):412-6.
[25] Passlick B, Born C, Haussinger K, Thetter O. Efficiency of video-assisted thoracic surgery for primary and secondary spontaneous pneumothorax. Ann Thorac Surg. 1998 Feb;65(2):324-7.

[26] Shaikhrezai K, Thompson AI, Parkin C, Stamenkovic S, Walker WS. Video-assisted thoracoscopic surgery management of spontaneous pneumothorax--long-term results. Eur J Cardiothorac Surg. 2011 Jul;40(1):120-3.

[27] Tanaka F, Itoh M, Esaki H, Isobe J, Ueno Y, Inoue R. Secondary spontaneous pneumothorax. Ann Thorac Surg. 1993 Feb;55(2):372-6.

[28] Lee SA, Sun JS, Park JH, Park KJ, Lee SS, Choi H, et al. Emphysema as a risk factor for the outcome of surgical resection of lung cancer. J Korean Med Sci. 2010 Aug;25(8):1146-51.

[29] Santambrogio L, Nosotti M, Baisi A, Ronzoni G, Bellaviti N, Rosso L. Pulmonary lobectomy for lung cancer: a prospective study to compare patients with forced expiratory volume in 1 s more or less than 80% of predicted. Eur J Cardiothorac Surg. 2001 Oct;20(4):684-7.

[30] Sekine Y, Behnia M, Fujisawa T. Impact of COPD on pulmonary complications and on long-term survival of patients undergoing surgery for NSCLC. Lung Cancer. 2002 Jul;37(1):95-101.

[31] Subotic DR, Mandaric DV, Eminovic TM, Gajic MM, Mujovic NM, Atanasijadis ND, et al. Influence of chronic obstructive pulmonary disease on postoperative lung function and complications in patients undergoing operations for primary non-small cell lung cancer. J Thorac Cardiovasc Surg. 2007 Nov;134(5):1292-9.

[32] Ciccone AM, Meyers BF, Guthrie TJ, Davis GE, Yusen RD, Lefrak SS, et al. Long-term outcome of bilateral lung volume reduction in 250 consecutive patients with emphysema. J Thorac Cardiovasc Surg. 2003 Mar;125(3):513-25.

[33] Lederer DJ, Thomashow BM, Ginsburg ME, Austin JH, Bartels MN, Yip CK, et al. Lung-volume reduction surgery for pulmonary emphysema: Improvement in body mass index, airflow obstruction, dyspnea, and exercise capacity index after 1 year. J Thorac Cardiovasc Surg. 2007 Jun;133(6):1434-8.

[34] Nicotera SP, Decamp MM. Special situations: air leak after lung volume reduction surgery and in ventilated patients. Thorac Surg Clin. 2010 Aug;20(3):427-34.

[35] Brunelli A, Varela G, Refai M, Jimenez MF, Pompili C, Sabbatini A, et al. A scoring system to predict the risk of prolonged air leak after lobectomy. Ann Thorac Surg. 2010 Jul;90(1):204-9.

[36] Cerfolio RJ, Bass CS, Pask AH, Katholi CR. Predictors and treatment of persistent air leaks. Ann Thorac Surg. 2002 Jun;73(6):1727-30; discussion 30-1.

[37] Isowa N, Hasegawa S, Bando T, Wada H. Preoperative risk factors for prolonged air leak following lobectomy or segmentectomy for primary lung cancer. Eur J Cardiothorac Surg. 2002 May;21(5):951.

[38] Lee L, Hanley SC, Robineau C, Sirois C, Mulder DS, Ferri LE. Estimating the risk of prolonged air leak after pulmonary resection using a simple scoring system. J Am Coll Surg. 2011 Jun;212(6):1027-32.

[39] Rivera C, Bernard A, Falcoz PE, Thomas P, Schmidt A, Benard S, et al. Characterization and prediction of prolonged air leak after pulmonary resection: a nationwide study setting up the index of prolonged air leak. Ann Thorac Surg. 2011 Sep;92(3):1062-8.

[40] Temes RT, Willms CD, Endara SA, Wernly JA. Fissureless lobectomy. Ann Thorac Surg. 1998 Jan;65(1):282-4.

[41] Nomori H, Ohtsuka T, Horio H, Naruke T, Suemasu K. Thoracoscopic lobectomy for lung cancer with a largely fused fissure. Chest. 2003 Feb;123(2):619-22.

[42] Gomez-Caro A, Calvo MJ, Lanzas JT, Chau R, Cascales P, Parrilla P. The approach of fused fissures with fissureless technique decreases the incidence of persistent air leak after lobectomy. Eur J Cardiothorac Surg. 2007 Feb;31(2):203-8.

[43] Ng T, Ryder BA, Machan JT, Cioffi WG. Decreasing the incidence of prolonged air leak after right upper lobectomy with the anterior fissureless technique. J Thorac Cardiovasc Surg. 2010 Apr;139(4):1007-11.

[44] Swanson SJ, Mentzer SJ, DeCamp MM, Jr., Bueno R, Richards WG, Ingenito EP, et al. No-cut thoracoscopic lung plication: a new technique for lung volume reduction surgery. J Am Coll Surg. 1997 Jul;185(1):25-32.

[45] Iwasaki M, Nishiumi N, Kaga K, Kanazawa M, Kuwahira I, Inoue H. Application of the fold plication method for unilateral lung volume reduction in pulmonary emphysema. Ann Thorac Surg. 1999 Mar;67(3):815-7.

[46] Mineo TC, Pompeo E, Mineo D, Tacconi F, Marino M, Sabato AF. Awake nonresectional lung volume reduction surgery. Ann Surg. 2006 Jan;243(1):131-6.

[47] Pompeo E, Mineo TC. Two-year improvement in multidimensional body mass index, airflow obstruction, dyspnea, and exercise capacity index after nonresectional lung volume reduction surgery in awake patients. Ann Thorac Surg. 2007 Dec;84(6):1862-9; discussion -9.

[48] Tacconi F, Pompeo E, Mineo TC. Duration of air leak is reduced after awake nonresectional lung volume reduction surgery. Eur J Cardiothorac Surg. 2009 May;35(5):822-8; discussion 8.

[49] Pompeo E, Rogliani P, Tacconi F, Dauri M, Saltini C, Novelli G, et al. Randomized comparison of awake nonresectional versus nonawake resectional lung volume reduction surgery. J Thorac Cardiovasc Surg. 2011 Nov 4.

[50] Pompeo E, Tacconi F, Mineo TC. Comparative results of non-resectional lung volume reduction performed by awake or non-awake anesthesia. Eur J Cardiothorac Surg. 2011 Apr;39(4):e51-8.

[51] Roberson LD, Netherland DE, Dhillon R, Heath BJ. Air leaks after surgical stapling in lung resection: a comparison between stapling alone and stapling with staple-line reinforcement materials in a canine model. J Thorac Cardiovasc Surg. 1998 Aug;116(2):353-4.

[52] Juettner FM, Kohek P, Pinter H, Klepp G, Friehs G. Reinforced staple line in severely emphysematous lungs. J Thorac Cardiovasc Surg. 1989 Mar;97(3):362-3.

[53] Miller JI, Jr., Landreneau RJ, Wright CE, Santucci TS, Sammons BH. A comparative study of buttressed versus nonbuttressed staple line in pulmonary resections. Ann Thorac Surg. 2001 Jan;71(1):319-22; discussion 23.

[54] Venuta F, Rendina EA, De Giacomo T, Flaishman I, Guarino E, Ciccone AM, et al. Technique to reduce air leaks after pulmonary lobectomy. Eur J Cardiothorac Surg. 1998 Apr;13(4):361-4.

[55] Hazelrigg SR, Boley TM, Naunheim KS, Magee MJ, Lawyer C, Henkle JQ, et al. Effect of bovine pericardial strips on air leak after stapled pulmonary resection. Ann Thorac Surg. 1997 Jun;63(6):1573-5.

[56] Stammberger U, Klepetko W, Stamatis G, Hamacher J, Schmid RA, Wisser W, et al. Buttressing the staple line in lung volume reduction surgery: a randomized three-center study. Ann Thorac Surg. 2000 Dec;70(6):1820-5.

[57] Fischel RJ, McKenna RJ, Jr. Bovine pericardium versus bovine collagen to buttress staples for lung reduction operations. Ann Thorac Surg. 1998 Jan;65(1):217-9.
[58] Baysungur V, Tezel C, Ergene G, Sevilgen G, Okur E, Uskul B, et al. The autologous pleural buttressing of staple lines in surgery for bullous lung disease. Eur J Cardiothorac Surg. 2010 Dec;38(6):679-82.
[59] Fleisher AG, Evans KG, Nelems B, Finley RJ. Effect of routine fibrin glue use on the duration of air leaks after lobectomy. Ann Thorac Surg. 1990 Jan;49(1):133-4.
[60] Wong K, Goldstraw P. Effect of fibrin glue in the reduction of postthoracotomy alveolar air leak. Ann Thorac Surg. 1997 Oct;64(4):979-81.
[61] Fabian T, Federico JA, Ponn RB. Fibrin glue in pulmonary resection: a prospective, randomized, blinded study. Ann Thorac Surg. 2003 May;75(5):1587-92.
[62] Moser C, Opitz I, Zhai W, Rousson V, Russi EW, Weder W, et al. Autologous fibrin sealant reduces the incidence of prolonged air leak and duration of chest tube drainage after lung volume reduction surgery: a prospective randomized blinded study. J Thorac Cardiovasc Surg. 2008 Oct;136(4):843-9.
[63] Porte HL, Jany T, Akkad R, Conti M, Gillet PA, Guidat A, et al. Randomized controlled trial of a synthetic sealant for preventing alveolar air leaks after lobectomy. Ann Thorac Surg. 2001 May;71(5):1618-22.
[64] Wain JC, Kaiser LR, Johnstone DW, Yang SC, Wright CD, Friedberg JS, et al. Trial of a novel synthetic sealant in preventing air leaks after lung resection. Ann Thorac Surg. 2001 May;71(5):1623-8; discussion 8-9.
[65] Allen MS, Wood DE, Hawkinson RW, Harpole DH, McKenna RJ, Walsh GL, et al. Prospective randomized study evaluating a biodegradable polymeric sealant for sealing intraoperative air leaks that occur during pulmonary resection. Ann Thorac Surg. 2004 May;77(5):1792-801.
[66] De Leyn P, Muller MR, Oosterhuis JW, Schmid T, Choong CK, Weder W, et al. Prospective European multicenter randomized trial of PleuraSeal for control of air leaks after elective pulmonary resection. J Thorac Cardiovasc Surg. 2011 Apr;141(4):881-7.
[67] Macchiarini P, Wain J, Almy S, Dartevelle P. Experimental and clinical evaluation of a new synthetic, absorbable sealant to reduce air leaks in thoracic operations. J Thorac Cardiovasc Surg. 1999 Apr;117(4):751-8.
[68] Venuta F, Diso D, De Giacomo T, Anile M, Rendina EA, Coloni GF. Use of a polymeric sealant to reduce air leaks after lobectomy. J Thorac Cardiovasc Surg. 2006 Aug;132(2):422-3.
[69] D'Andrilli A, Andreetti C, Ibrahim M, Ciccone AM, Venuta F, Mansmann U, et al. A prospective randomized study to assess the efficacy of a surgical sealant to treat air leaks in lung surgery. Eur J Cardiothorac Surg. 2009 May;35(5):817-20; discussion 20-1.
[70] Tan C, Utley M, Paschalides C, Pilling J, Robb JD, Harrison-Phipps KM, et al. A prospective randomized controlled study to assess the effectiveness of CoSeal(R) to seal air leaks in lung surgery. Eur J Cardiothorac Surg. 2011 Aug;40(2):304-8.
[71] Lang G, Csekeo A, Stamatis G, Lampl L, Hagman L, Marta GM, et al. Efficacy and safety of topical application of human fibrinogen/thrombin-coated collagen patch (TachoComb) for treatment of air leakage after standard lobectomy. Eur J Cardiothorac Surg. 2004 Feb;25(2):160-6.

[72] Anegg U, Lindenmann J, Matzi V, Smolle J, Maier A, Smolle-Juttner F. Efficiency of fleece-bound sealing (TachoSil) of air leaks in lung surgery: a prospective randomised trial. Eur J Cardiothorac Surg. 2007 Feb;31(2):198-202.

[73] Rena O, Papalia E, Mineo TC, Massera F, Pirondini E, Turello D, et al. Air-leak management after upper lobectomy in patients with fused fissure and chronic obstructive pulmonary disease: a pilot trial comparing sealant and standard treatment. Interact Cardiovasc Thorac Surg. 2009 Dec;9(6):973-7.

[74] Belda-Sanchis J, Serra-Mitjans M, Iglesias Sentis M, Rami R. Surgical sealant for preventing air leaks after pulmonary resections in patients with lung cancer. Cochrane Database Syst Rev. 2010(1):CD003051.

[75] Belcher E, Dusmet M, Jordan S, Ladas G, Lim E, Goldstraw P. A prospective, randomized trial comparing BioGlue and Vivostat for the control of alveolar air leak. J Thorac Cardiovasc Surg. 2010 Jul;140(1):32-8.

[76] Tansley P, Al-Mulhim F, Lim E, Ladas G, Goldstraw P. A prospective, randomized, controlled trial of the effectiveness of BioGlue in treating alveolar air leaks. J Thorac Cardiovasc Surg. 2006 Jul;132(1):105-12.

[77] Brunelli A, Al Refai M, Monteverde M, Borri A, Salati M, Sabbatini A, et al. Pleural tent after upper lobectomy: a randomized study of efficacy and duration of effect. Ann Thorac Surg. 2002 Dec;74(6):1958-62.

[78] Allama AM. Pleural tent for decreasing air leak following upper lobectomy: a prospective randomised trial. Eur J Cardiothorac Surg. 2010 Dec;38(6):674-8.

[79] Okur E, Kir A, Halezeroglu S, Alpay AL, Atasalihi A. Pleural tenting following upper lobectomies or bilobectomies of the lung to prevent residual air space and prolonged air leak. Eur J Cardiothorac Surg. 2001 Nov;20(5):1012-5.

[80] Cerfolio RJ, Holman WL, Katholi CR. Pneumoperitoneum after concomitant resection of the right middle and lower lobes (bilobectomy). Ann Thorac Surg. 2000 Sep;70(3):942-6; discussion 6-7.

[81] Handy JR, Jr., Judson MA, Zellner JL. Pneumoperitoneum to treat air leaks and spaces after a lung volume reduction operation. Ann Thorac Surg. 1997 Dec;64(6):1803-5.

[82] De Giacomo T, Rendina EA, Venuta F, Francioni F, Moretti M, Pugliese F, et al. Pneumoperitoneum for the management of pleural air space problems associated with major pulmonary resections. Ann Thorac Surg. 2001 Nov;72(5):1716-9.

[83] Korasidis S, Andreetti C, D'Andrilli A, Ibrahim M, Ciccone A, Poggi C, et al. Management of residual pleural space and air leaks after major pulmonary resection. Interact Cardiovasc Thorac Surg. 2010 Jun;10(6):923-5.

[84] Clavero JM, Cheyre JE, Solovera ME, Aparicio RP. Transient diaphragmatic paralysis by continuous para-phrenic infusion of bupivacaine: a novel technique for the management of residual spaces. Ann Thorac Surg. 2007 Mar;83(3):1216-8.

[85] Hollaus PH, Lax F, Janakiev D, Lucciarini P, Katz E, Kreuzer A, et al. Endoscopic treatment of postoperative bronchopleural fistula: experience with 45 cases. Ann Thorac Surg. 1998 Sep;66(3):923-7.

[86] Scappaticci E, Ardissone F, Ruffini E, Baldi S, Revello F, Coni F. As originally published in 1994: Postoperative bronchopleural fistula: endoscopic closure in 12 patients. Updated in 2000. Ann Thorac Surg. 2000 May;69(5):1629-30.

[87] Varoli F, Roviaro G, Grignani F, Vergani C, Maciocco M, Rebuffat C. Endoscopic treatment of bronchopleural fistulas. Ann Thorac Surg. 1998 Mar;65(3):807-9.

[88] Martin WR, Siefkin AD, Allen R. Closure of a bronchopleural fistula with bronchoscopic instillation of tetracycline. Chest. 1991 Apr;99(4):1040-2.
[89] Ponn RB, D'Agostino RS, Stern H, Westcott JL. Treatment of peripheral bronchopleural fistulas with endobronchial occlusion coils. Ann Thorac Surg. 1993 Dec;56(6):1343-7.
[90] Sprung J, Krasna MJ, Yun A, Thomas P, Bourke DL. Treatment of a bronchopleural fistula with a Fogarty catheter and oxidized regenerated cellulose (surgicel). Chest. 1994 Jun;105(6):1879-81.
[91] Jones DP, David I. Gelfoam occlusion of peripheral bronchopleural fistulas. Ann Thorac Surg. 1986 Sep;42(3):334-5.
[92] Watanabe S, Shimokawa S, Yotsumoto G, Sakasegawa K. The use of a Dumon stent for the treatment of a bronchopleural fistula. Ann Thorac Surg. 2001 Jul;72(1):276-8.
[93] Kramer MR, Peled N, Shitrit D, Atar E, Saute M, Shlomi D, et al. Use of Amplatzer device for endobronchial closure of bronchopleural fistulas. Chest. 2008 Jun;133(6):1481-4.
[94] Kiriyama M, Fujii Y, Yamakawa Y, Fukai I, Yano M, Kaji M, et al. Endobronchial neodymium:yttrium-aluminum garnet laser for noninvasive closure of small proximal bronchopleural fistula after lung resection. Ann Thorac Surg. 2002 Mar;73(3):945-8; discussion 8-9.
[95] West D, Togo A, Kirk AJ. Are bronchoscopic approaches to post-pneumonectomy bronchopleural fistula an effective alternative to repeat thoracotomy? Interact Cardiovasc Thorac Surg. 2007 Aug;6(4):547-50.
[96] Mitchell KM, Boley TM, Hazelrigg SR. Endobronchial valves for treatment of bronchopleural fistula. Ann Thorac Surg. 2006 Mar;81(3):1129-31.
[97] Feller-Kopman D, Bechara R, Garland R, Ernst A, Ashiku S. Use of a removable endobronchial valve for the treatment of bronchopleural fistula. Chest. 2006 Jul;130(1):273-5.
[98] Travaline JM, McKenna RJ, Jr., De Giacomo T, Venuta F, Hazelrigg SR, Boomer M, et al. Treatment of persistent pulmonary air leaks using endobronchial valves. Chest. 2009 Aug;136(2):355-60.
[99] Gillespie CT, Sterman DH, Cerfolio RJ, Nader D, Mulligan MS, Mularski RA, et al. Endobronchial valve treatment for prolonged air leaks of the lung: a case series. Ann Thorac Surg. 2011 Jan;91(1):270-3.
[100] Andersen I, Nissen H. Results of silver nitrate pleurodesis in spontaneous pneumothorax. Dis Chest. 1968 Sep;54(3):230-3.
[101] Janzing HM, Derom A, Derom E, Eeckhout C, Derom F, Rosseel MT. Intrapleural quinacrine instillation for recurrent pneumothorax or persistent air leak. Ann Thorac Surg. 1993 Feb;55(2):368-71.
[102] Chen JS, Hsu HH, Chen RJ, Kuo SW, Huang PM, Tsai PR, et al. Additional minocycline pleurodesis after thoracoscopic surgery for primary spontaneous pneumothorax. Am J Respir Crit Care Med. 2006 Mar 1;173(5):548-54.
[103] Almassi GH, Haasler GB. Chemical pleurodesis in the presence of persistent air leak. Ann Thorac Surg. 1989 May;47(5):786-7.
[104] Read CA, Reddy VD, O'Mara TE, Richardson MS. Doxycycline pleurodesis for pneumothorax in patients with AIDS. Chest. 1994 Mar;105(3):823-5.

[105] Balassoulis G, Sichletidis L, Spyratos D, Chloros D, Zarogoulidis K, Kontakiotis T, et al. Efficacy and safety of erythromycin as sclerosing agent in patients with recurrent malignant pleural effusion. Am J Clin Oncol. 2008 Aug;31(4):384-9.
[106] Patz EF, Jr., McAdams HP, Erasmus JJ, Goodman PC, Culhane DK, Gilkeson RC, et al. Sclerotherapy for malignant pleural effusions: a prospective randomized trial of bleomycin vs doxycycline with small-bore catheter drainage. Chest. 1998 May;113(5):1305-11.
[107] Olivares-Torres CA, Laniado-Laborin R, Chavez-Garcia C, Leon-Gastelum C, Reyes-Escamilla A, Light RW. Iodopovidone pleurodesis for recurrent pleural effusions. Chest. 2002 Aug;122(2):581-3.
[108] Rivas de Andres JJ, Blanco S, de la Torre M. Postsurgical pleurodesis with autologous blood in patients with persistent air leak. Ann Thorac Surg. 2000 Jul;70(1):270-2.
[109] Lang-Lazdunski L, Coonar AS. A prospective study of autologous 'blood patch' pleurodesis for persistent air leak after pulmonary resection. Eur J Cardiothorac Surg. 2004 Nov;26(5):897-900.
[110] Droghetti A, Schiavini A, Muriana P, Comel A, De Donno G, Beccaria M, et al. Autologous blood patch in persistent air leaks after pulmonary resection. J Thorac Cardiovasc Surg. 2006 Sep;132(3):556-9.
[111] Shackcloth M, Poullis M, Page R. Autologous blood pleurodesis for treating persistent air leak after lung resection. Ann Thorac Surg. 2001 Apr;71(4):1402-3.
[112] Brant A, Eaton T. Serious complications with talc slurry pleurodesis. Respirology. 2001 Sep;6(3):181-5.
[113] Kuzniar TJ, Blum MG, Kasibowska-Kuzniar K, Mutlu GM. Predictors of acute lung injury and severe hypoxemia in patients undergoing operative talc pleurodesis. Ann Thorac Surg. 2006 Dec;82(6):1976-81.
[114] Baron RD, Milton R, Thorpe JA. Pleurodesis using small talc particles results in an unacceptably high rate of acute lung injury and hypoxia. Ann Thorac Surg. 2007 Dec;84(6):2136.
[115] Shaw P, Agarwal R. Pleurodesis for malignant pleural effusions. Cochrane Database Syst Rev. 2004(1):CD002916.
[116] Cooper JD, Patterson GA, Sundaresan RS, Trulock EP, Yusen RD, Pohl MS, et al. Results of 150 consecutive bilateral lung volume reduction procedures in patients with severe emphysema. J Thorac Cardiovasc Surg. 1996 Nov;112(5):1319-29; discussion 29-30.
[117] Ayed AK. Suction versus water seal after thoracoscopy for primary spontaneous pneumothorax: prospective randomized study. Ann Thorac Surg. 2003 May;75(5):1593-6.
[118] Cerfolio RJ, Bass C, Katholi CR. Prospective randomized trial compares suction versus water seal for air leaks. Ann Thorac Surg. 2001 May;71(5):1613-7.
[119] Marshall MB, Deeb ME, Bleier JI, Kucharczuk JC, Friedberg JS, Kaiser LR, et al. Suction vs water seal after pulmonary resection: a randomized prospective study. Chest. 2002 Mar;121(3):831-5.
[120] Brunelli A, Monteverde M, Borri A, Salati M, Marasco RD, Al Refai M, et al. Comparison of water seal and suction after pulmonary lobectomy: a prospective, randomized trial. Ann Thorac Surg. 2004 Jun;77(6):1932-7; discussion 7.

[121] Brunelli A, Sabbatini A, Xiume F, Refai MA, Salati M, Marasco R. Alternate suction reduces prolonged air leak after pulmonary lobectomy: a randomized comparison versus water seal. Ann Thorac Surg. 2005 Sep;80(3):1052-5.

[122] Alphonso N, Tan C, Utley M, Cameron R, Dussek J, Lang-Lazdunski L, et al. A prospective randomized controlled trial of suction versus non-suction to the under-water seal drains following lung resection. Eur J Cardiothorac Surg. 2005 Mar;27(3):391-4.

[123] Ponn RB, Silverman HJ, Federico JA. Outpatient chest tube management. Ann Thorac Surg. 1997 Nov;64(5):1437-40.

[124] McKenna RJ, Jr., Fischel RJ, Brenner M, Gelb AF. Use of the Heimlich valve to shorten hospital stay after lung reduction surgery for emphysema. Ann Thorac Surg. 1996 Apr;61(4):1115-7.

[125] Rieger KM, Wroblewski HA, Brooks JA, Hammoud ZT, Kesler KA. Postoperative outpatient chest tube management: initial experience with a new portable system. Ann Thorac Surg. 2007 Aug;84(2):630-2.

[126] Cerfolio RJ, Minnich DJ, Bryant AS. The removal of chest tubes despite an air leak or a pneumothorax. Ann Thorac Surg. 2009 Jun;87(6):1690-4; discussion 4-6.

[127] Suter M, Bettschart V, Vandoni RE, Cuttat JF. Thoracoscopic pleurodesis for prolonged (or intractable) air leak after lung resection. Eur J Cardiothorac Surg. 1997 Jul;12(1):160-1.

[128] Stefani A, Jouni R, Alifano M, Bobbio A, Strano S, Magdeleinat P, et al. Thoracoplasty in the current practice of thoracic surgery: a single-institution 10-year experience. Ann Thorac Surg. 2011 Jan;91(1):263-8.

[129] Woo E, Tan BK, Lim CH. Treatment of recalcitrant air leaks: the combined latissimus dorsi-serratus anterior flap. Ann Plast Surg. 2009 Aug;63(2):188-92.

[130] Chee CB, Abisheganaden J, Yeo JK, Lee P, Huan PY, Poh SC, et al. Persistent air-leak in spontaneous pneumothorax--clinical course and outcome. Respir Med. 1998 May;92(5):757-61.

[131] Michaels BM, Orgill DP, Decamp MM, Pribaz JJ, Eriksson E, Swanson S. Flap closure of postpneumonectomy empyema. Plast Reconstr Surg. 1997 Feb;99(2):437-42.

[132] Abolhoda A, Bui TD, Milliken JC, Wirth GA. Pedicled latissimus dorsi muscle flap: routine use in high-risk thoracic surgery. Tex Heart Inst J. 2009;36(4):298-302.

[133] Jiang L, Jiang GN, He WX, Fan J, Zhou YM, Gao W, et al. Free rectus abdominis musculocutaneous flap for chronic postoperative empyema. Ann Thorac Surg. 2008 Jun;85(6):2147-9.

[134] Watanabe H, Imaizumi M, Takeuchi S, Murase M, Hasegawa T. Treatment of empyema by transposition of contralateral lower trapezius flap. Ann Thorac Surg. 1997 Mar;63(3):837-9.